Synthesis Lectures on Biomedical Engineering

This series consists of concise books on advanced and state-of-the-art topics that span the field of biomedical engineering. Each Lecture covers the fundamental principles in a unified manner, develops underlying concepts needed for sequential material, and progresses to more advanced topics and design. The authors selected to write the Lectures are leading experts on the subject who have extensive background in theory, application, and design. The series is designed to meet the demands of the 21st century technology and the rapid advancements in the all-encompassing field of biomedical engineering

Rohit Thanki

AI Role in Haptic Healthcare

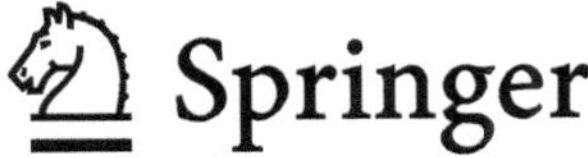

Rohit Thanki
Senior IEEE Member
Rajkot, Gujarat, India

ISSN 1930-0328   ISSN 1930-0336   (electronic)
Synthesis Lectures on Biomedical Engineering
ISBN 978-3-032-24906-7   ISBN 978-3-032-24907-4   (eBook)
https://doi.org/10.1007/978-3-032-24907-4

This Springer imprint is published by the registered company Springer Nature Switzerland AG
The registered company address is: Gewerbestrasse 11, 6330 Cham, Switzerland

If disposing of this product, please recycle the paper.

Preface

The convergence of artificial intelligence (AI) and haptic technologies is reshaping the landscape of modern healthcare, offering unprecedented opportunities to enhance patient care, surgical precision, rehabilitation, and medical education. This book, *AI Roles in Haptic Healthcare*, provides a comprehensive exploration of this transformative field, bridging the gap between theoretical foundations, clinical applications, and future innovations.

The journey begins with an introduction to the historical evolution of medical technology, setting the stage for understanding how AI and haptics are revolutionizing healthcare. From robotic surgery to smart prosthetics, telemedicine, and pain management, the book delves into the diverse applications of AI-powered haptic systems, showcasing their ability to restore tactile feedback, improve patient outcomes, and expand access to care. The book also addresses the critical challenges that must be overcome to ensure the responsible deployment of these technologies. It examines the ethical implications of AI-mediated medical decisions, the need for robust data privacy and security measures, and the importance of mitigating algorithmic bias. Furthermore, it highlights the safety-critical nature of haptic devices and the rigorous engineering and regulatory standards required for their clinical use.

Looking ahead, the book explores emerging technologies such as mid-air haptics, neuromorphic chips, and brain-computer interfaces, which promise to redefine the boundaries of tactile medicine. It envisions a future where AI-haptic systems are seamlessly integrated into smart hospital ecosystems, enabling personalized medicine through patient digital twins and multi-omics data. The book also outlines a research and innovation roadmap, emphasizing the need for global collaboration, open science, and equitable access to ensure that these advancements benefit all of humanity.

This book is intended for researchers, clinicians, engineers, policymakers, and anyone interested in the transformative potential of AI and haptics in healthcare. It is both a technical guide and a call to action, urging stakeholders to embrace responsible innovation and ethical stewardship as we navigate the exciting yet complex future of AI-driven haptic healthcare.

By synthesizing cutting-edge research, real-world applications, and visionary insights, *AI Role in Haptic Healthcare* aims to inspire and equip readers to contribute to this rapidly evolving field. Together, we can create a future where technology enhances human touch, restores lost sensations, and extends the reach of skilled care to every corner of the globe.

Rajkot, India   Rohit Thanki

Acknowledgments

Our task has been made easier and the final version of this book considerably improved thanks to the support we have received. We extend our heartfelt thanks to the publishing team for their invaluable guidance and encouragement during the creation of this book. We also wish to thank our colleagues and peers for their insightful discussions and contributions that enriched the content.

Competing Interests The author has no competing interests to declare that are relevant to the content of this manuscript.

Contents

List of Tables

Introduction to AI and Haptic Technologies in Healthcare

1

This chapter establishes the foundational framework for understanding the transformative convergence of artificial intelligence (AI) and haptic technologies in modern healthcare. Beginning with the historical evolution of medical technology, the chapter systematically examines the role of AI in contemporary medicine, the scientific principles underlying haptic feedback systems, the clinical importance of tactile information, and the emerging applications that arise when these two powerful technology streams are combined. The chapter concludes by critically assessing the adoption landscape including regulatory, technical, and clinical challenges while highlighting the profound opportunities these innovations present for patient care, surgical precision, and medical education.

The evolution of technology in healthcare has progressed through several distinct phases, beginning with analog imaging modalities such as X-rays and mechanical instruments, advancing to digital innovations like computed tomography (CT), magnetic resonance imaging (MRI), and electronic health records, and culminating in the present era of AI-driven platforms that leverage complex algorithms for diagnostic and predictive tasks. Key artificial intelligence techniques now applied in modern medicine include deep learning, which excels in pattern recognition for medical imaging and genomics, and reinforcement learning, which is used to optimize treatment protocols and robotic control. At the same time, an understanding of the biophysical mechanisms underlying the human sense of touch such as mechanoreceptors, neural pathways, and tactile perception is crucial for the development of medical haptics, which simulate touch and force feedback in clinical environments. Major haptic technology types include tactile displays, force-feedback devices, and wearable sensors, each serving specific clinical applications such as minimally invasive surgery, rehabilitation, and remote diagnosis. The convergence of AI and haptic systems is enabled by architectures that integrate AI perception, prediction, and control with haptic output, creating interactive platforms for enhanced medical decision-making and procedural accuracy. However, the adoption of AI-haptic systems in

R. Thanki, *AI Role in Haptic Healthcare*, Synthesis Lectures on Biomedical Engineering, https://doi.org/10.1007/978-3-032-24907-4_1

1

healthcare faces ongoing challenges related to regulatory compliance, technical integration, and clinical validation, while also presenting profound opportunities to improve patient care, surgical precision, and medical education.

1.1   Evolution of Technology in Healthcare

Healthcare has always been shaped by the technological capabilities of its era. The discovery of X-rays by Wilhelm Rontgen in 1895 marked the first major step toward non-invasive internal visualization, fundamentally altering diagnostic practice. However, the pace of technological adoption remained gradual through most of the twentieth century. The true acceleration began in the 1970s with the advent of computed tomography (CT) and magnetic resonance imaging (MRI), which enabled clinicians to visualize soft tissue anatomy with unprecedented clarity [1].

The 1990s introduced the digital revolution into clinical workflows. Electronic Health Record (HER) systems replaced paper-based documentation, enabling longitudinal patient data to be accessed, shared, and analysed. The parallel rise of the internet created the infrastructure for telemedicine, allowing specialist consultations to cross geographic boundaries. These developments set the stage for what would become one of the most consequential shifts in the history of medicine: the entry of artificial intelligence. From 2005 onward, machine learning algorithms began demonstrating performance comparable to domain experts in narrow but high-stakes tasks, such as classifying diabetic retinopathy from retinal fundus images [2]. By 2015, the integration of AI with physical interaction systems, robotics and haptics began emerging as a distinct and rapidly maturing field. Table 1.1 presents a structured overview of these developmental phases. Figure 1.1 shows a timeline of key technological transitions in healthcare, from analog imaging to AI-haptic convergence.

What distinguishes the current era is not merely technological sophistication but systemic integration. AI does not simply add computational speed; it enables systems that

Table 1.1 Phases of technology evolution in healthcare

Era	Period	Key technology	Impact on healthcare
Pre-digital	Before 1970	Mechanical instruments, X-rays, ECG	Standardized diagnostics
Digital Dawn	1970–1990	CT/MRI scanners, electronic records	Imaging revolution
Information	1990–2005	EHR systems, telemedicine, internet	Connectivity and data sharing
AI emergence	2005–2015	Machine learning in radiology and genomics	Pattern recognition at scale
AI-haptic fusion	2015–present	Robot-assisted surgery, VR/AR simulation	Precision and tactile intelligence
Future vision	2025+	Autonomous surgical robots, neuro-haptics	Personalized and remote care

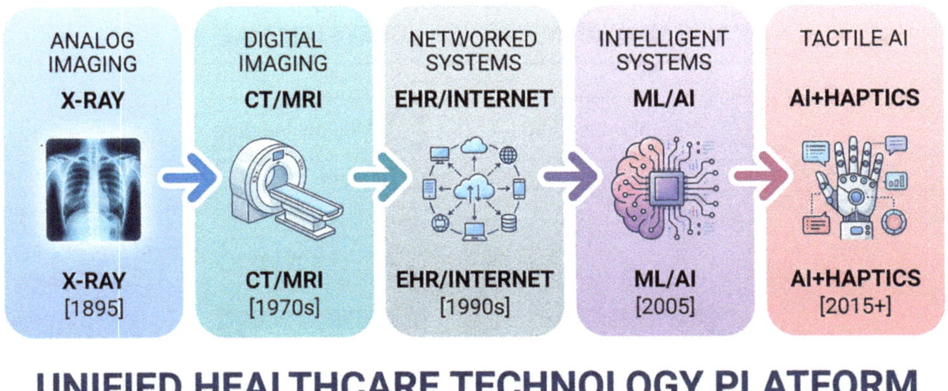

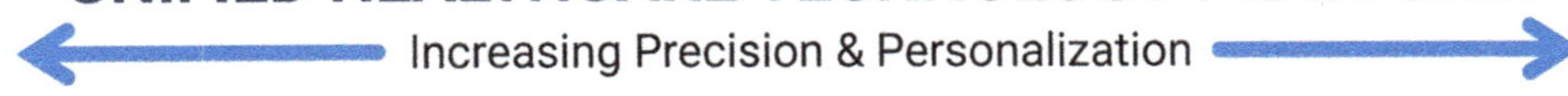

Fig. 1.1 Timeline of key technological transitions in healthcare

perceive, reason, and adapt qualities that, when coupled with haptic feedback capable of simulating physical touch, create fundamentally new categories of medical capability [1, 2].

1.2   Role of Artificial Intelligence in Modern Medicine

Artificial intelligence, broadly defined as the capacity of machines to perform tasks that would otherwise require human intelligence, encompasses a spectrum of techniques including machine learning, deep learning, natural language processing (NLP), computer vision, and reinforcement learning. In the medical domain, these tools address a fundamental challenge: the exponential growth of clinical data has far outpaced human capacity for analysis [1].

Deep learning, particularly convolutional neural networks (CNNs), has demonstrated transformative potential in medical imaging. Google DeepMind's AI system for detecting over 50 eye diseases from optical coherence tomography (OCT) scans matched the diagnostic accuracy of leading ophthalmologists, while processing each scan in under 30 s [1]. Similarly, AI-driven analysis of whole-slide pathology images has shown concordance with expert pathologists in cancer grading tasks [2].

Beyond imaging, NLP-based systems extract clinically relevant information from unstructured physician notes, enabling cohort analyses that were previously impossible. Reinforcement learning (RL) is increasingly applied in surgical robotics and drug dosing optimization domains where sequential decision-making under uncertainty is critical [3]. Federated learning architectures allow multiple hospital systems to train shared AI models without exposing patient data directly, addressing GDPR and HIPAA concerns [4]. Figure 1.2 shows the AI ecosystem in modern healthcare systems while Table 1.2 gives core AI techniques and their applications in healthcare.

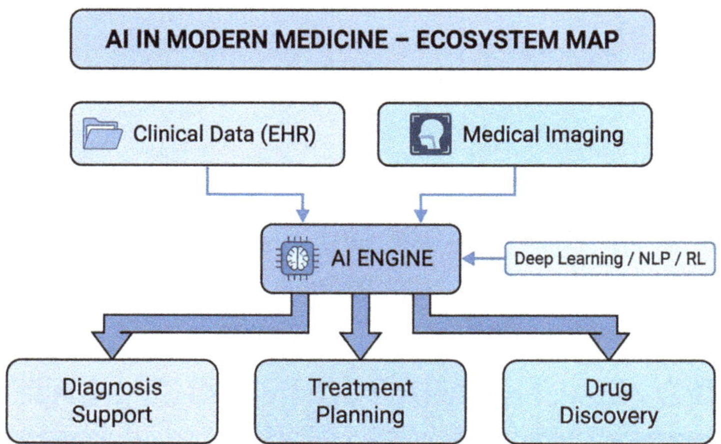

Fig. 1.2 AI ecosystem in modern medicine

Table 1.2 Core AI techniques and their medical applications

AI technique	Core capability	Medical application	Example system
Deep learning (CNNs)	Image feature extraction	Radiology, pathology	Google DeepMind (eye disease)
Reinforcement learning	Adaptive decision-making	Surgical robotics	OpenAI dexterous hand
Natural language processing	Clinical text understanding	EHR summarization	GPT-4 in clinical notes
Computer vision	Real-time scene analysis	Laparoscopic guidance	Intuitive da Vinci
Federated learning	Privacy-preserving training	Multi-hospital AI	NVIDIA FLARE platform
Generative AI	Synthetic data creation	Rare disease simulation	Synthea, DALL-E med
Graph neural networks	Relational data analysis	Drug discovery	AlphaFold2 (DeepMind)

The regulatory dimension of AI in medicine is increasingly formalized. In the European Union, AI-enabled medical devices are classified as Software as a Medical Device (SaMD) under EU MDR 2017/745, requiring clinical evidence, post-market surveillance, and conformity assessment proportional to risk classification (Class I–III). The U.S. FDA has published a proposed regulatory framework for AI/ML-based SaMD that accommodates iterative model updates [4]. These frameworks will directly govern the deployment of AI-haptic systems.

1.3   Understanding Haptic Technology and the Science of Touch

Haptics, derived from the Greek haptikos, meaning 'able to touch', refers to the science and technology of simulating the sense of touch through forces, vibrations, and motions applied to the user. To engineer effective haptic systems, a thorough understanding of the biological substrate of touch is essential.

1.3.1   The Somatosensory System

Human skin contains four principal classes of mechanoreceptors; each tuned to distinct physical stimuli. Merkel discs (SA-I) respond to sustained pressure and spatial form; Meissner corpuscles (RA-I) detect light touch and object slip during manipulation; Ruffini endings (SA-II) encode skin stretch and finger position; and Pacinian corpuscles (RA-II) are exquisitely sensitive to high-frequency vibrations (40–400 Hz), critical for detecting surface textures during tool mediated exploration [5]. These signals are transmitted via large diameter myelinated afferent fibres (Aβ) to the primary somatosensory cortex (S1), where spatiotemporal patterns are decoded into perceptual experience.

Understanding the frequency-response characteristics and spatial acuity of each receptor type is directly related to haptic device design [5, 6]. For instance, vibrotactile actuators used in surgical gloves must operate within the frequency range most effectively detected by Pacinian corpuscles to convey meaningful texture information. Figure 1.3 shows the tactile receptor types of somatosensory in human skin and their respective stimulus sensitivities.

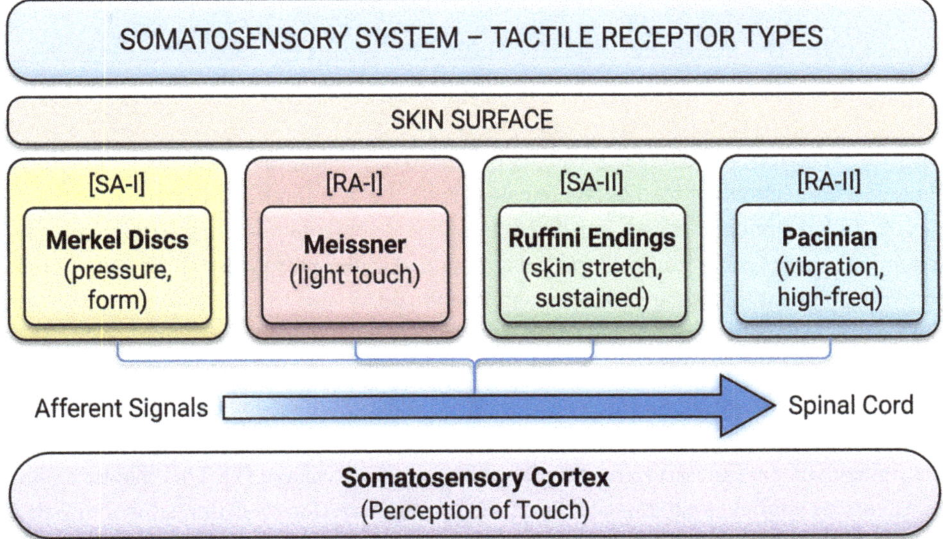

Fig. 1.3 Somatosensory receptor types in human skin and their respective stimulus sensitivities

Table 1.3 Haptic technology types, mechanisms, and medical applications

Type	Mechanism	Sensation delivered	Medical use case
Vibrotactile	Vibrating motors/actuators	Texture, vibration	Surgical training simulators
Force feedback	Motorized resistance	Stiffness, resistance	Robotic surgery (da Vinci)
Electro tactile	Electrical skin stimulation	Tingling, pressure	Prosthetic limb feedback
Thermal haptics	Thermoelectric modules	Heat, cold	Burn wound assessment
Pneumatic	Air pressure chambers	Pressure, inflation	Minimally invasive tools
Ultrasonic mid-air	Focused ultrasound waves	Contactless pressure	Touchless UI in OR
Neuro-direct	Neural interfaces	Complex sensations	BCI prosthetics (research)

1.3.2 Haptic Technology Modalities

Haptic systems are broadly classified into three categories: tactile (cutaneous) feedback systems that act on the skin surface; kinaesthetic (proprioceptive) systems that convey forces and joint positions through muscles and tendons; and combined systems that integrate both [6]. Table 1.3 provides a comprehensive taxonomy of haptic modalities relevant to medical applications.

Force-feedback systems, exemplified by the Geomagic Touch and Phantom Premium devices, allow surgeons and trainees to feel tissue resistance, suture tension, and needle puncture forces during simulation [7]. Vibrotactile arrays embedded in surgical gloves or tool handles can encode texture and surface compliance information from robotic instruments. Emerging mid-air haptic systems using focused ultrasound enable gesture-based control of sterile OR environments without physical contact — a significant advantage given infection control requirement [6].

1.4   Importance of Touch in Medical Practice

Physical palpation, the clinical act of feeling tissues, organs, and anatomical structures, remains a cornerstone of medical diagnosis despite the proliferation of imaging technologies. A skilled clinician's hands can detect lymph node enlargement, hepatosplenomegaly, abdominal masses, skin lesion characteristics, and vascular pulsatility with a level of integrative judgement that imaging alone cannot replicate.

In surgical practice, tactile feedback is even more critical. Laparoscopic and robotic minimally invasive surgeries inherently attenuate or eliminate the tactile information surgeons receive through direct instrument-tissue contact. Studies consistently demonstrate that reduced haptic feedback in robotic surgery correlates with increased risk of inadvertent tissue damage, excessive grasping force, and suture breakage [7]. This 'haptic deficit' represents a significant patient safety concern, particularly for procedures involving delicate structures such as bile ducts, neural tissue, and vascular anastomoses.

Beyond surgery, touch plays a crucial therapeutic role. Manual physical therapy, osteopathic manipulation, neonatal care, and wound assessment all depend fundamentally on the clinician's tactile skills. The ageing global population and increasing prevalence of chronic pain conditions have heightened demand for rehabilitative technologies that can provide calibrated, reproducible tactile stimulation, a gap that AI-driven haptic rehabilitation platforms are beginning to address [8].

1.5   Convergence of AI and Haptic Systems

The convergence of AI and haptic technologies represents a paradigm shift from passive sensing and output to active, intelligent, closed-loop interaction. In classical haptic systems, feedback is deterministic: a predefined force profile is triggered by sensor readings according to hard-coded rules. AI transforms this paradigm by enabling the system to learn, predict, and adapt based on accumulated experience [9].

Consider a robotic surgical assistant equipped with AI-haptic integration. As the robot's instrument contacts tissue, embedded force and tactile sensors capture multi-axis interaction data. A deep learning model trained on thousands of annotated surgical recordings classifies the contacted tissue type (e.g. healthy parenchyma vs. tumour margin vs. vascular structure) in real time. A reinforcement learning controller then modulates the force feedback rendered to the surgeon's hand controllers, amplifying sensations at critical tissue boundaries while suppressing irrelevant mechanical noise [10]. Simultaneously, a predictive model anticipates tissue deformation under applied forces, allowing the system to provide anticipatory haptic cues before the surgeon's instruments physically contact sensitive structures.

Figure 1.4 shows the architecture of the AI-haptic system for healthcare. This architecture shows that sensing input → perception AI → prediction AI → control AI → haptic output represents the general framework applicable across surgical robotics, rehabilitation, telemedicine, and simulation. The feedback loop must operate at latencies below 1 ms to avoid perceptual instability, placing extreme demands on edge computing infrastructure [9]. From a regulatory standpoint, AI-haptic systems that directly influence surgical decision-making are likely to be classified as Class IIb or Class III medical devices under EU MDR, requiring notified body assessment [4].

1.6   Overview of AI-Driven Haptic Healthcare Applications

The application landscape for AI-haptic healthcare systems is rapidly diversifying across four primary domains: surgical robotics, medical simulation and training, physical rehabilitation, and remote examination. Figure 1.5 shows the applications of AI-driven haptic healthcare system.

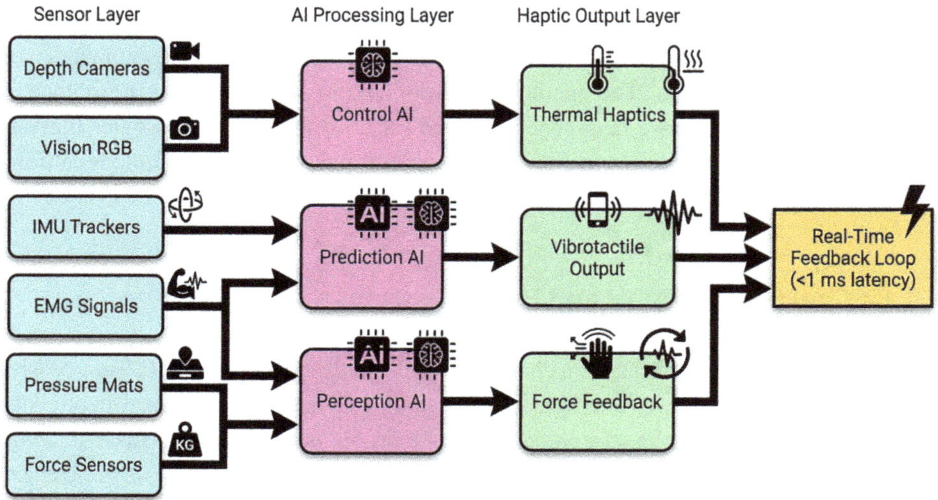

Fig. 1.4 AI-haptic convergence architecture showing the sensing, AI processing, and haptic output pipeline with a real-time feedback loop

1.6.1   Surgical Robotics

Robotic surgical platforms such as Intuitive Surgical's da Vinci system have demonstrated measurable clinical benefits including reduced blood loss, shorter hospital stays, and faster patient recovery [11]. However, the current generation of surgical robots provides limited or no haptic feedback to the operating surgeon. Next-generation platforms incorporating AI-driven haptic restoration aim to address this limitation. Research prototypes have demonstrated that AI-predicted force feedback can approach the perceptual fidelity of direct tissue palpation [12].

1.6.2   Medical Simulation and Training

High-fidelity haptic simulators are transforming procedural skills training. Systems such as the Simbionix LAP Mentor and Fundamental Surgery VR platform combine physics-based tissue models with AI-generated patient-specific tissue properties derived from pre-operative imaging [13]. Performance analytics provided by embedded AI assess force application patterns, instrument trajectory efficiency, and error rates, providing objective, reproducible skill metrics that traditional apprenticeship models cannot offer.

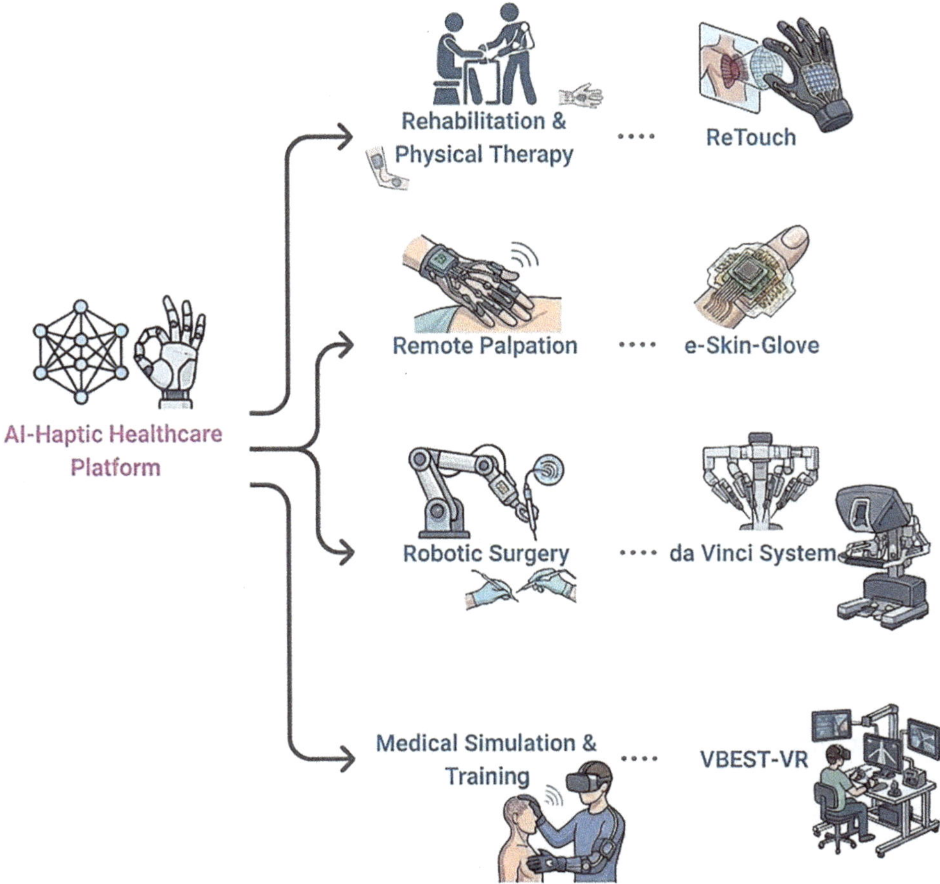

Fig. 1.5 Overview of AI-driven haptic healthcare application domains—from robotic surgery to remote palpation

1.6.3 Physical Rehabilitation

Stroke rehabilitation and musculoskeletal recovery benefit significantly from haptic-assisted therapy. Robotic exoskeletons such as the Hocoma Armeo and ReWalk system deliver calibrated assistive or resistive forces during movement rehabilitation. AI models trained on patient movement data dynamically adjust assistance levels, providing more support during fatigued movement phases and progressively withdrawing assistance as motor function recovers [8].

1.6.4   Remote Palpation and Telemedicine

Perhaps the most ambitious application domain is remote palpation, enabling a clinician to physically examine a patient located thousands of kilometres away. The landmark transatlantic Lindbergh Operation in 2001 demonstrated the conceptual feasibility of teleoperated surgery [14]. AI-haptic teleoperation systems address the fundamental challenge of communication latency: predictive AI models generate local haptic responses that anticipate the remote tissue's reaction, masking network delays below the perceptual threshold [10].

1.7   Opportunities and Challenges in Adoption

The clinical translation of AI-haptic systems confronts a multidimensional adoption landscape that spans technical, regulatory, economic, human factors, and ethical dimensions. Table 1.4 shows the challenges and mitigation strategies for AI adoption in the healthcare sector.

1.7.1   Technical Challenges

The most fundamental technical constraint is latency. The human haptic system detects timing discrepancies as small as 1 ms; force-feedback loops must therefore operate at update rates exceeding 1 kHz to maintain perceptual stability. Achieving this in wireless, teleoperated environments demands edge computing infrastructure co-located with robotic systems [9]. Sensor miniaturization, particularly for tri-axial force and tactile sensor arrays that can be integrated into minimally invasive surgical instruments, remains an active area

Table 1.4 AI-haptic adoption challenges and mitigation strategies

Challenge	Category	Mitigation strategy	Current status
Latency (<1 ms required)	Technical	Edge computing, 5G	Active R&D
Regulatory approval (EU MDR)	Regulatory	SaMD classification pathway	Complex but navigable
High development cost	Financial	Modular platform design	Barrier for SMEs
Interoperability gaps	Technical	FHIR/HL7 integration	Standards emerging
Clinical validation burden	Clinical	RCT & real-world evidence	Required for CE mark
Surgeon adoption resistance	Human factors	Training & simulation programs	Improving
AI model explainability	Regulatory/ ethical	XAI frameworks	Growing tooling
Data privacy (GDPR)	Legal	Federated/on-device AI	Technically viable

of materials science research. Data fusion across heterogeneous sensor modalities (force, vision, EMG, temperature) requires AI architectures capable of real-time multi-modal processing with deterministic timing guarantees [9].

1.7.2   Regulatory Pathway

In the European Union, AI-haptic surgical systems will typically be classified as Class IIb or III SaMD under EU MDR 2017/745, requiring a full clinical investigation demonstrating safety and performance [4]. The integration of adaptive AI, where models update based on accumulated real-world data requires transparent change management documentation and ongoing post-market clinical follow-up (PMCF). Developers must also address ISO 13485:2016 quality management requirements, IEC 62304 software lifecycle standards, and increasingly, ISO/IEC 42001 for AI management systems.

1.7.3   Economic and Market Access Considerations

The capital expenditure for AI-haptic surgical platforms currently ranging from $1.5 M to $2 M per installation limits adoption to large academic medical centres and well-funded private hospital networks [15]. Health technology assessment (HTA) bodies require health-economic evidence demonstrating cost-effectiveness over standard of care. Innovative reimbursement models including procedure-based bundled payments, AI-as-a-service subscription structures, and outcome-linked pricing are being explored to democratize access.

1.7.4   Human Factors and Clinical Adoption

Even technically superior systems face adoption barriers rooted in workflow integration and user acceptance [13]. Explainable AI (XAI) frameworks that provide surgeons with interpretable rationales for AI-driven haptic cues rather than simply asserting 'danger ahead' are essential for building clinical trust. Simulation-based training curricula must be developed in parallel with device deployment to ensure practitioners can exploit the full capability of these systems safely [4].

1.7.5   Ethical and Privacy Dimensions

AI-haptic systems that acquire detailed biomechanical data during surgical procedures raise significant data governance questions. Under GDPR and sector-specific health data regulations, patient consent frameworks must address secondary data use for AI model training [4]. Bias in AI models trained predominantly on data from high-income healthcare settings may result in systems that perform sub-optimally on underrepresented patient populations, a health equity concern requiring proactive attention in dataset curation strategies [4].

1.8   Summary

This chapter examines the multifaceted considerations involved in the development and deployment of AI-haptic surgical systems. Regulatory requirements under the EU MDR 2017/745 mandate that these systems, often classified as Class IIb or III SaMD, undergo rigorous clinical investigation and continuous post-market monitoring, with strict adherence to standards such as ISO 13485:2016, IEC 62304, and ISO/IEC 42001 for AI management. Economic barriers are notable, as high capital costs currently restrict access to major academic and private hospital networks, prompting exploration of innovative reimbursement models like bundled payments and AI-as-a-service subscriptions.

Human factors are equally critical; clinical adoption hinges on integrating explainable AI to foster user trust and developing simulation-based training to maximize safe and effective use. Ethical and privacy dimensions are underscored by the need for robust data governance under GDPR, informed patient consent for secondary data use, and the mitigation of bias through diverse and representative datasets. Collectively, these elements highlight the importance of a holistic approach that addresses regulatory, economic, human, and ethical challenges to advance equitable and safe adoption of AI-haptic surgical technologies.

References

1. Topol, E. J. (2019). High-performance medicine: The convergence of human and artificial intelligence. *Nature Medicine, 25*(1), 44–56. https://doi.org/10.1038/s41591-018-0300-7
2. Esteva, A., Kuprel, B., Novoa, R. A., Ko, J., Swetter, S. M., Blau, H. M., & Thrun, S. (2017). Dermatologist-level classification of skin cancer with deep neural networks. *Nature, 542*(7639), 115–118. https://doi.org/10.1038/nature21056
3. Yip, M., & Das, N. (2019). Robot autonomy for surgery. In *The encyclopedia of medical robotics: Vol. 1. Minimally invasive surgical robotics* (pp. 281–313).
4. World Health Organization. (2021). *Ethics and governance of artificial intelligence for health.* World Health Organization.
5. Johansson, R. S., & Flanagan, J. R. (2009). Coding and use of tactile signals from the fingertips in object manipulation tasks. *Nature Reviews Neuroscience, 10*(5), 345–359. https://doi.org/10.1038/nrn2621
6. Pacchierotti, C., Sinclair, S., Solazzi, M., Frisoli, A., Hayward, V., & Prattichizzo, D. (2017). Wearable haptic systems for the fingertip and the hand: Taxonomy, review, and perspectives. *IEEE Transactions on Haptics, 10*(4), 580–600.

7. Okamura, A. M. (2009). Haptic feedback in robot-assisted minimally invasive surgery. *Current Opinion in Urology, 19*(1), 102–107.

8. Shanmugam, M., Venusamy, K., Subin, S., Srivatsan, S., & Kumar, N. (2023, March). A comprehensive review of haptic gloves: Advances, challenges, and future directions. In *2023 Second International Conference on Electronics and Renewable Systems (ICEARS)* (pp. 227–233). IEEE.

9. Tiwari, G., Kumar, S., Tiwari, N., & Cengiz, K. (2025). Technical challenges and innovations in AI-enhanced haptic systems for healthcare. In *Integrating AI with haptic systems for Smarter Healthcare Solutions* (pp. 27–46). IGI Global Scientific Publishing.

10. Badhan, A. K., Bhattacharjee, A., Kumar, R., & Diwan, P. (2025). Machine learning algorithms for adaptive haptic responses. In *Integrating AI with haptic systems for Smarter Healthcare Solutions* (pp. 199–232). IGI Global Scientific Publishing.

11. Zemmar, A., Lozano, A. M., & Nelson, B. J. (2020). The rise of robots in surgical environments during COVID-19. *Nature Machine Intelligence, 2*(10), 566–572.

12. El Rassi, I., & El Rassi, J. M. (2020). A review of haptic feedback in tele-operated robotic surgery. *Journal of Medical Engineering & Technology, 44*(5), 247–254.

13. Riek, L. D. (2017). Healthcare robotics. *Communications of the ACM, 60*(11), 68–78.

14. Marescaux, J., Leroy, J., Gagner, M., Rubino, F., Mutter, D., Vix, M., et al. (2001). Transatlantic robot-assisted telesurgery. *Nature, 413*(6854), 379–380.

15. Global Robotic Surgery Market Size (2025–2032). *Growth of minimally invasive and AI-powered surgery, trends, competitive landscape, regional outlook, and opportunities with AI-enabled surgical systems.* Retrieved January 2026, from https://www.mmrstatistics.com/reports/795456/global-robotic-surgery-market

Fundamentals of Artificial Intelligence and Haptic Systems

2

This chapter provides a rigorous technical foundation in both artificial intelligence and haptic systems as they apply to healthcare. The chapter begins by establishing core AI and machine learning concepts, progresses through deep learning architectures and their clinical deployments, and then transitions to the biophysics and engineering principles underpinning haptic feedback. Hardware components such as sensors, actuators, and wearable devices are systematically examined, culminating in detailed treatment of the AI algorithms specifically engineered to process and act on haptic data streams. By the end of this chapter, readers will possess the conceptual vocabulary and technical grounding necessary to understand the integrated AI-haptic systems examined in subsequent chapters.

Artificial intelligence (AI) refers to the broad field of computer science focused on developing systems capable of performing tasks that typically require human intelligence, such as reasoning, perception, and decision-making. Within AI, machine learning (ML) is a subset that enables computers to learn from data and improve performance over time without being explicitly programmed. Deep learning, a further specialization of ML, utilizes multi-layered neural networks to automatically extract features from large datasets, allowing for sophisticated pattern recognition and predictive modelling. These paradigms are interrelated: deep learning models are a type of machine learning, which in turn are foundational to artificial intelligence. In medical contexts, supervised learning is used for tasks like disease diagnosis, where labelled data (e.g. annotated medical images) guide the model; unsupervised learning helps uncover hidden patterns in patient records or genomic data without predefined labels; and reinforcement learning optimizes treatment protocols or robotic control via trial-and-error feedback in dynamic environments. Key deep learning architectures include convolutional neural networks (CNNs) for medical image analysis, long short-term memory (LSTM) networks for interpreting sequential patient data, Transformers for natural language processing in electronic health records, and U-Net models for biomedical image segmentation. Haptic feedback operates on the principle of

R. Thanki, *AI Role in Haptic Healthcare*, Synthesis Lectures on Biomedical Engineering, https://doi.org/10.1007/978-3-032-24907-4_2

providing tactile or force sensations to users, often within a closed-loop system architecture where sensors detect user interactions, actuators deliver physical feedback, and AI algorithms adjust outputs in real time. Haptic technologies are classified by modality—such as tactile displays, force-feedback devices, and wearable sensors—with applications ranging from minimally invasive surgery to rehabilitation and remote diagnostics. The hardware backbone of haptic systems comprises sensors that capture touch and force data, actuators that generate feedback, and wearable devices that interface directly with clinicians or patients. Advanced AI algorithms process haptic data streams for signal classification and predictive rendering, enabling responsive, interactive experiences that enhance procedural accuracy and medical decision-making.

2.1   Basics of Artificial Intelligence and Machine Learning

Artificial intelligence (AI) is the branch of computer science concerned with building systems that exhibit behaviours typically associated with human cognition such as perception, reasoning, learning, planning, and language understanding. Machine learning (ML) is the dominant sub-discipline of AI, characterized by algorithms that improve their performance on a task through exposure to data rather than through explicit programming [1, 2]. This distinction is foundational: whereas a traditional rule-based system for detecting cardiac arrhythmias requires cardiologists to codify every decision boundary, an ML system learns those boundaries automatically from thousands of annotated electrocardiograms. Figure 2.1 shows the hierarchical relationship between AI, machine learning, and deep learning sub-fields.

2.1.1   The Machine Learning Landscape

Machine learning paradigms differ principally in the nature of the supervisory signal available during training [2]. In supervised learning, every training example carries a ground-truth label; the algorithm minimizes a loss function measuring the discrepancy between its prediction and the label. In unsupervised learning, no labels are provided; the algorithm must discover latent structure, clusters, manifolds, or generative factors within the data. Reinforcement occupies a distinct position: an agent interacts with an environment, receiving scalar reward signals, and learning a policy that maximizes cumulative future reward. Table 2.1 provides a structured comparison of the major ML paradigms with healthcare illustrations.

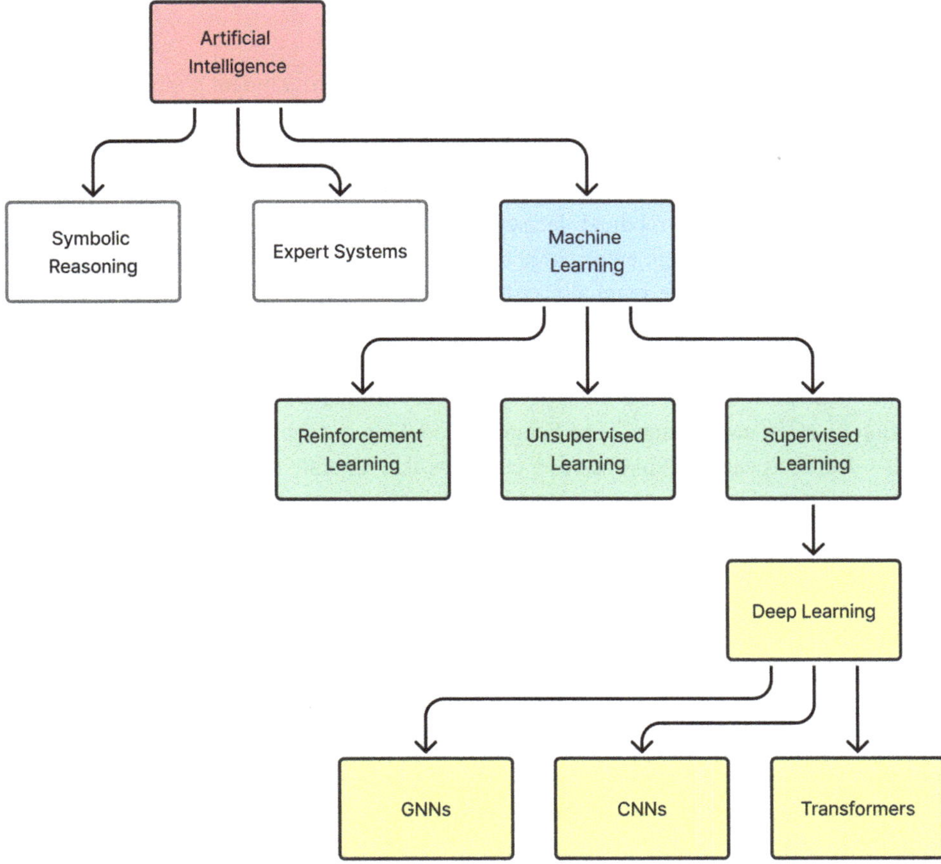

Fig. 2.1 Taxonomy of artificial intelligence

Table 2.1 Machine learning paradigms, characteristics, and healthcare applications

Paradigm	Learning mode	Core technique	Healthcare example
Supervised	Labelled data	CNN, SVM, Logistic Regression	Tumour classification from MRI
Unsupervised	Unlabelled data	K-Means, Autoencoders, PCA	Patient phenotyping, anomaly detection
Semi-supervised	Partial labels	Self-training, Label Propagation	EHR representation learning
Reinforcement	Reward signals	Q-Learning, PPO, DDPG	Adaptive drug dosing, surgical robotics
Self-supervised	Contrastive objectives	SimCLR, DINO, MAE	Pre-training on unlabelled scans
Federated	Distributed data	FedAvg, Fed Prox	Multi-hospital privacy-preserving AI

2.1.2 Key Concepts in Machine Learning

Several concepts are central to understanding ML systems in clinical contexts. The bias-variance trade-off describes the tension between a model's ability to fit training data (low bias) and its ability to generalize to unseen patients (low variance) [2]. Overfitting where a model memorizestraining examples rather than learning generalizable patterns is a persistent risk when labelled medical datasets are small. Regularization techniques (L1/L2 penalties, dropout, data augmentation) and cross-validation are standard mitigations.

Feature engineering, the manual construction of informative input representations, is the dominant bottleneck in classical ML. Deep learning largely supersedes hand-crafted features by learning hierarchical representations directly from raw inputs [1]. This is of value in medical imaging, where the pixel-level discriminative features encoding tumour morphology resist easy manual specification. Model interpretability, the degree to which a model's decisions can be explained to a clinician, is a separate and increasingly regulated concern, addressed through explainable AI (XAI) techniques such as SHAP values, LIME, and gradient-weighted class activation maps (Grad-CAM).

2.2 Deep Learning in Healthcare Applications

Deep learning refers to a class of machine learning models comprising multiple layers of parameterited, differentiable transformations, collectively capable of learning arbitrarily complex input-output mappings from data [1]. The seminal demonstration that deep convolutional networks could surpass human performance in large-scale visual recognition (ImageNet, 2012) catalysed an explosion of healthcare applications. Simultaneously, advances in graphics processing unit (GPU) hardware, automatic differentiation frameworks (TensorFlow, PyTorch), and the availability of large annotated medical datasets created the conditions for rapid translation. Figure 2.2 shows a generic deep learning pipeline in healthcare which gives raw clinical input through preprocessing, model inference, to structured clinical output. Table 2.2 shows various deep learning architectures and their healthcare applications.

2.2.1 Convolutional Neural Networks (CNNs)

CNNs exploit the spatial structure of images through local receptive fields, weight sharing across spatial locations, and hierarchical feature abstraction. Early convolutional layers detect low-level features (edges, gradients); deeper layers encode semantic structures (lesion boundaries, tissue texture patterns) [1, 3]. In medical imaging, CNNs have achieved regulatory clearance or breakthrough device designation from the FDA for applications including diabetic retinopathy screening, pulmonary nodule detection, and stroke triage on non-contrast CT. A critical architectural extension is the U-Net [4], originally developed

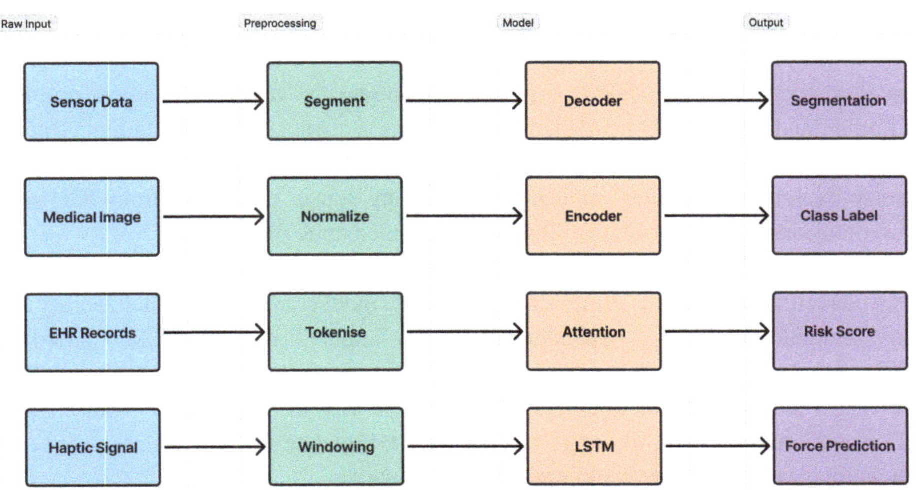

Fig. 2.2 Generic deep learning pipeline in healthcare

Table 2.2 Deep learning architectures and their healthcare applications

Architecture	Key feature	Input type	Medical application
CNN	Spatial feature maps	Images, video	Radiology, pathology, dermatology
RNN/LSTM	Sequence memory	Time series, text	ECG analysis, clinical notes NLP
Transformer	Self-attention	Text, images, multi-modal	Report generation, drug interaction
U-Net	Encoder-decoder + skip	Medical images	Tumour and organ segmentation
GAN	Generative adversarial	Images	Synthetic training data, augmentation
Graph NN	Relational structures	Molecular graphs, EHR	Drug discovery, comorbidity mapping
Diffusion models	Iterative denoising	Images	Medical image synthesis, denoising

for biomedical image segmentation. U-Net introduces skip connections between encoder and decoder pathways, allowing the network to combine high-resolution spatial information with deep semantic representations. This property is indispensable for precise tumour delineation on MRI and CT, organ-at-risk contouring in radiotherapy planning, and retinal vessel segmentation for diabetic screening.

2.2.2 Recurrent Architectures and Transformers

Long short-term memory (LSTM) networks [5] address the vanishing gradient problem that limits standard recurrent neural networks on long sequences. LSTMs maintain a gated cell state that selectively retains or discards information over hundreds of time steps, a property exploited in clinical applications including sepsis prediction from ICU time series, medication adherence modelling, and real-time haptic prediction.

The Transformer architecture [6], introduced with the self-attention mechanism, has displaced recurrent models as the dominant sequence model due to its parallelizability and ability to model long-range dependencies. Large language models (LLMs) based on Transformer decoders underpin clinical NLP applications including automated radiology report generation, discharge summary synthesis, and ICD coding. Vision Transformers (ViT) extend self-attention to image patches, achieving state-of-the-art performance on medical image classification with large training corpora.

2.2.3 Federated and Self-Supervised Learning

Federated learning [7] addresses the fundamental tension between AI training data requirements and patient privacy regulations (GDPR, HIPAA). Rather than centralizing patient data, federated frameworks train local model copies at each participating hospital and aggregate only gradient updates or model weights at a central server. The NVIDIA FLARE platform and Google's federated learning toolkit have been deployed in multi-institutional cancer imaging studies, enabling model training across hundreds of thousands of cases while maintaining data locality.

Self-supervised learning pre-trains models on unlabelled medical data by constructing proxy tasks predicting masked image patches, contrasting augmented views of the same scan before fine-tuning on small, labelled datasets [3]. This approach is particularly valuable in healthcare, where expert annotation is expensive and scarce. Foundation models pre-trained on millions of unlabelled radiographs, pathology slides, or clinical notes can be fine-tuned to new tasks with as few as dozens of labelled examples.

2.3 Fundamentals of Haptic Feedback and Tactile Interfaces

Haptic systems are human–machine interfaces that communicate information through the sense of touch by applying forces, vibrations, or displacements to the user's body. The engineering challenge is formidable: the human somatosensory system is sensitive to temporal events as brief as 1 ms, spatial features as small as 1 mm, and force magnitudes spanning five orders of magnitude from the threshold of perception (~0.01 N) to safe maximum gripping forces [8]. Haptic systems must match this dynamic range while maintaining stability in closed-loop interaction. Figure 2.3 shows the architecture of a haptic

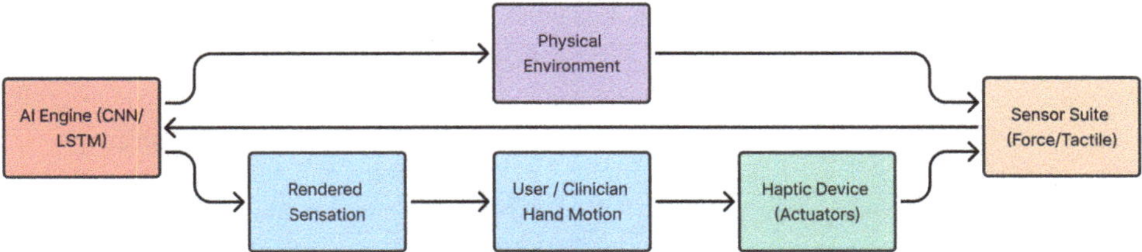

Fig. 2.3 Closed-loop architecture of a haptic feedback system

feedback system that has the bidirectional flow between the user, haptic device, sensor suite, AI engine, and physical environment.

2.3.1 The Haptic Rendering Loop

The fundamental computational architecture of a haptic system is the rendering loop, a high-rate (typically 500 Hz to 2 kHz) closed-loop control cycle that [7, 9]: (1) reads position and force sensors; (2) computes a virtual environment model (deformation, contact, friction); (3) determines the haptic feedback force or texture; and (4) commands the actuators. The requirement for deterministic timing within 1 ms places haptic rendering in the category of hard real-time computing, necessitating dedicated processor cores, real-time operating systems, and hardware interrupt-driven I/O.

Stability is the central concern in haptic system design. When a haptic device interacts with a stiff virtual surface, the combination of actuator dynamics, rendering delay, and sensing noise can produce unstable force oscillations, a phenomenon known as haptic wall penetration or chattering. Z-width, defined as the range of impedances a haptic display can stably and transparently render, is the primary performance metric for kinaesthetic devices [9]. AI-based adaptive controllers can dynamically adjust rendering parameters to maintain stability across varying interaction scenarios.

The modalities outlined in Table 2.3 highlight the diverse range of haptic feedback mechanisms employed in advanced systems to simulate realistic touch sensations. Kinaesthetic feedback focuses on the perception of force, torque, and position, which is essential for tasks requiring precision and resistance, such as surgical procedures or robotic grasping. On the other hand, vibrotactile feedback is crucial for conveying information about texture and vibrations, enabling users to detect surface irregularities and slippage. Together, these modalities support a wide spectrum of clinical and practical applications, enhancing user interaction with physical environments through more natural and intuitive feedback.

Table 2.3 Diverse range of haptic feedback modalities

Category	Sensation	Frequency range	Clinical relevance
Kinaesthetic	Force, torque, position	DC–50 Hz	Surgical resistance, grasping force
Vibrotactile	Texture, vibration	20–1000 Hz	Surface texture, slip detection
Thermal	Temperature gradients	0.01–5 Hz	Tissue inflammation, burn assessment
Electrotactile	Electrical nerve stimulation	1–500 Hz	Prosthetic limb sensation
Pneumatic	Pressure, inflation	0.1–20 Hz	Tissue distension in MIS
Mid-air ultrasonic	Focused acoustic radiation	40 kHz carrier	Touchless OR interface control

2.3.2 Deformable Body Simulation for Medical Haptics

Realistic haptic rendering of biological tissue requires accurate real-time simulation of soft body deformation. Classical approaches use the Finite Element Method (FEM) to solve the equations of solid mechanics; however, standard FEM is computationally too slow for haptic rates. Reduced-order modelling, pre-computed deformation modes, and GPU-accelerated FEM solvers have brought real-time tissue simulation to haptic rates for moderate mesh densities [10]. Physics-informed neural networks [11] embed partial differential equations governing tissue mechanics directly into the network training objective, enabling fast inference of deformation fields with physical consistency guarantees, a promising direction for patient-specific haptic simulation.

2.4   Types of Haptic Technologies

Haptic technologies are classified according to the type of sensation they deliver, the actuation principle employed, and the body region to which feedback is applied. Each modality presents a distinct trade-off between fidelity, bandwidth, wearability, and suitability for sterile clinical environments [12, 13]. Figure 2.4 provides a structured overview of haptic technology varieties as they relate to specific clinical applications, highlighting the importance of matching the type of sensations such as prosthetic touch, thermal sense, or touchless interface with the fidelity demanded in medical environments. By categorizing technologies like thermoelectric wound assessment, mid-air ultrasonic sterile interactions, and MEMS-based AR-guided procedures, the figure underscores how each approach is tailored to unique requirements ranging from tactile feedback in prosthetics to precise, sterile controls in operating theatres. This mapping facilitates informed selection and integration of haptic solutions, ensuring that medical devices effectively support clinical outcomes and patient safety by delivering appropriate sensory feedback and interaction modes.

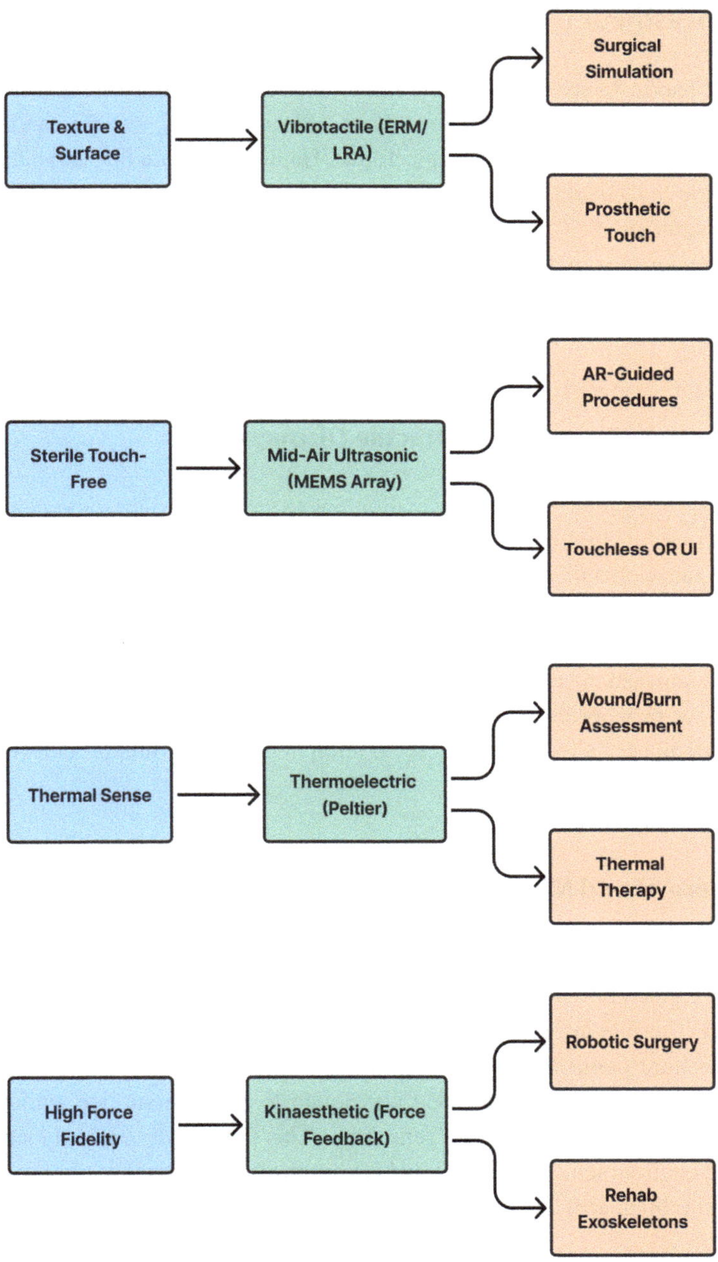

Fig. 2.4 Types of haptic technologies in clinical domain

2.4.1   Kinaesthetic (Force Feedback) Systems

Kinaesthetic haptic devices apply forces and torques to the joints and tendons of the user's hand or limb, conveying information about object stiffness, weight, and resistance. Grounded devices such as the Geomagic Touch, Haption Virtuose 6D, and delta.x parallel robots provide high-fidelity multi-axis force feedback with workspace volumes suitable for surgical simulation [9]. Ungrounded (wearable) exoskeletons such as the HaptX DK2 gloves use tendon-driven actuated joints to constrain finger motion, enabling the perception of object shape and stiffness in fully immersive virtual reality surgical training environments.

2.4.2   Vibrotactile and Electrotactile Displays

Vibrotactile devices deliver mechanical vibrations to the skin surface via eccentric rotating mass (ERM) motors or linear resonant actuators (LRAs). These actuators are compact, low-power, and well-suited for integration into wearable surgical gloves. Piezoelectric bimorph arrays enable spatial control of vibration patterns across the fingertip at frequencies up to 1 kHz [12]. Electrotactile stimulation bypasses mechanical actuation by delivering charge-controlled electrical pulses to cutaneous nerve fibres through electrode arrays on the skin surface, producing sensations of pressure, texture, and proprioception, a modality particularly suited to sensory restoration in upper limb amputees using myoelectric prostheses.

2.4.3   Thermal and Mid-Air Haptic Systems

Thermal haptic devices, based on Peltier thermoelectric elements, can rapidly modulate skin surface temperature to convey heat (vasodilation, inflammation) or cold (ischaemia, cryotherapy). Thermal information is diagnostically relevant in wound assessment, where tissue temperature gradients indicate vascular perfusion and infection boundaries [12]. Mid-air haptic systems project focused ultrasound to the skin surface without physical contact, producing localized pressure sensations. This modality is uniquely suited to sterile operating environments, enabling touchless control of OR displays, intraoperative AR overlays, and robotic arm commanding without contaminating the sterile field.

2.5 Hardware Components of Haptic Systems

A haptic system is an integration of mechanical, electrical, computational, and software subsystems. Understanding each component's contribution to overall system performance, bandwidth, force range, latency, and stability is essential for designing medical-grade devices that meet the stringent requirements of clinical and surgical environments [12, 13].

Table 2.4 provides an overview of the essential hardware components used in haptic systems, highlighting their types, key specifications, and representative platforms. Force-feedback arms utilize kinaesthetic actuators such as Geomagic Touch and Haption Virtuose, offering high-resolution six degrees of freedom (6-DOF) force control critical for medical and surgical applications. Vibrotactile arrays, employing ERM and LRA motors, deliver precise mechanical vibrations across a wide frequency range with minimal latency, as seen in devices like BioTac SP and SynTouch. These components illustrate the integration of advanced actuator technologies and real-time control electronics needed to achieve accurate, responsive, and safe haptic feedback in clinical environments.

2.5.1 Actuator Technologies

Electric motors such as brushed DC, brushless DC (BLDC), and stepper remain the dominant actuation principle for kinaesthetic haptic devices due to their high-power density, controllability, and back drivability (the ability to be moved by external forces with minimal resistance). Back drivability is critical: a non-back drivable actuator that fails creates a rigid mechanical barrier, posing a patient safety risk in surgical applications. Series elastic actuators (SEA) deliberately introduce a compliant spring element between the motor and output, improving force control fidelity and intrinsic mechanical safety at the cost of bandwidth [9].

Table 2.4 Types, specifications, and examples for hardware components of haptic systems

Component	Type	Key specification	Example/Platform
Force-feedback arm	Kinaesthetic actuator	6-DOF, 0.03 N resolution	Geomagic Touch, Haption Virtuose
Vibrotactile array	ERM/LRA motors	30–300 Hz, <1 ms latency	BioTac SP, SynTouch
Surgical robot end-effector	Multi-DOF manipulator	Sub-mm positioning	da Vinci EndoWrist, Hugo
Exoskeleton glove	Wearable kinaesthetic	10-DOF per hand	HaptX Gloves, CyberGrasp
Tactile display	Pin-array/shape memory	2 mm spatial resolution	KGS DotView, Metec B11
Thermal module	Peltier thermoelectric	±30 °C in <0.5 s	ThermoReal, ThermoWrist
Ultrasonic mid-air	MEMS phased array	40 kHz, 10 cm range	Ultrahaptics STRATOS

Pneumatic actuators are used in soft haptic gloves and surgical tool simulators where compliance and anatomical conformation are priorities over high bandwidth. Dielectric elastomer actuators (DEAs) and shape memory alloy (SMA) wires offer miniaturization advantages for implantable or catheter-mounted haptic elements, though their nonlinear dynamics require specialized AI-based controllers [7].

2.5.2   Control Electronics and Real-Time Computing

Haptic control loops execute at 1–2 kHz on real-time processors. The National Instruments CompactRIO, BeagleBone AI-64, and FPGA-based custom hardware are common platforms for deterministic haptic control. Field programmable gate arrays (FPGAs) are particularly well-suited because they implement control algorithms in dedicated digital logic with sub-microsecond determinism, eliminating operating system jitters. Communication between the haptic controller and the AI inference server typically uses EtherCAT or PCIe with latencies in the 100–500 μs range, ensuring the AI prediction does not introduce perceptible delay into the haptic loop [10].

2.6   Sensors, Actuators, and Wearable Devices

Sensors are the perceptual front-end of haptic systems, converting physical interactions between instrument and tissue (or hand and virtual object) into digital signals available for AI processing. The accuracy, bandwidth, and noise characteristics of sensors directly limit the realism and safety of haptic feedback [8, 12]. Table 2.5 summarizes key sensor technologies utilized in haptic systems, highlighting their measured parameters and clinical applications. Force/torque sensors, commonly based on strain gauge and MEMS technology, measure multidimensional forces and moments, enabling precise detection of tissue

Table 2.5 Sensor types for haptic systems

Sensor type	Measured parameter	Technology	Haptic system role
Force/torque	3-axis force and moment	Strain gauge, MEMS	Tissue contact force in robotic MIS
Tactile array	Pressure distribution	Capacitive, piezoresistive	Finger pad contact mapping
IMU	Orientation, acceleration	MEMS gyro + accel	Limb tracking in exoskeletons
EMG	Muscle activation	Surface electrode array	Intent detection for prosthetics
Optical encoder	Angular position	Rotary encoder disk	Kinaesthetic feedback calibration
Depth camera	3D geometry	Structured light/ToF	Tissue surface reconstruction
Flex sensor	Joint bending angle	Resistive film	Glove-based hand poses tracking

contact forces in robotic minimally invasive surgery. Tactile sensor arrays, utilizing capacitive or piezoresistive mechanisms, provide detailed pressure distribution data across contact surfaces, supporting finger pad contact mapping for enhanced realism and control. Together, these sensors form the foundation for accurate and responsive haptic feedback, playing essential roles in both clinical procedures and advanced training environments.

2.6.1   Force and Tactile Sensors

Six-axis force/torque (F/T) sensors are standard in robotic surgical tools and haptic research platforms. These devices use strain gauge Wheatstone bridge circuits etched into a compliant metallic structure to measure forces and moments along three orthogonal axes simultaneously. Commercial medical-grade F/T sensors (ATI Nano17, OptoForce) achieve force resolutions below 0.01 N with bandwidths exceeding 2 kHz, matching haptic rendering loop requirements [9]. Tactile sensor arrays provide spatially resolved pressure maps across the contact area. BioTac SP sensors (SynTouch) integrate fluid-filled elastic skin over an array of impedance electrodes and a hydrophone, enabling simultaneous measurement of normal force, shear force, vibration, temperature, and thermal flux, the richest multi-modal tactile data set currently available from a fingertip-sized sensor [8].

2.6.2   Wearable Haptic Devices

Wearable haptic devices integrate sensing and actuation in body-worn form factors, enabling untethered clinical and training applications [13]. The principal design challenges are: (1) power autonomy, active haptic actuation consumes significant power, limiting wireless operation to 2–4 h without inductive charging; (2) weight and ergonomics, devices on the finger or hand must not fatigue the user or impair natural dexterity; and (3) biocompatibility, materials in contact with skin must be hypoallergenic and sterilizable. State-of-the-art wearable haptic gloves, such as HaptX DK2 and Dextarobotics DEX, integrate pneumatic finger flexion resistance with vibrotactile arrays on each fingertip, providing a rich multi-modal experience for surgical simulation and remote palpation training [13]. Soft robotic finger thimbles using pneumatic microchannels are emerging as lightweight alternatives, achieving gripping force simulation up to 20 N within a form factor weighing under 30 g.

2.7   AI Algorithms for Haptic Data Processing

The integration of AI into haptic systems transforms their capability from static, preprogrammed responses to adaptive, context-aware haptic communication. AI algorithms in haptic systems fulfil four principal functions: perception (classifying the tissue or surface being touched), prediction (forecasting future states to compensate for latency), generation (synthesizing realistic haptic signals for simulation), and control (computing optimal actuator commands) [7, 10].

Figure 2.5 illustrates the comprehensive AI-driven workflow for haptic data processing in medical systems, beginning with the acquisition of multi-modal sensor inputs such as force/torque measurements, tactile arrays, and inertial data. These raw signals undergo essential preprocessing to extract relevant features and ensure data quality before entering the AI inference engine, which encompasses modules for tissue classification, force prediction, deformation modelling, and safety monitoring. The intelligent algorithms process these features to deliver precise, context-aware outputs, which are then translated into real-time actuator commands via haptic rendering with sub-millisecond latency. This tightly integrated pipeline enables responsive and safe tactile feedback in clinical applications, bridging the gap between advanced sensing and immediate force feedback for medical interventions.

Table 2.6 summarizes the diverse roles played by advanced AI algorithms in modern haptic systems. Techniques such as one-dimensional convolutional neural networks (1D CNNs) are employed for classifying force time series data, enabling accurate tissue type recognition crucial for surgical and diagnostic applications. Long Short-Term Memory (LSTM) models, on the other hand, handle sequence prediction tasks by processing streams from various sensors, thereby supporting predictive force rendering to overcome latency issues in teleoperation. By leveraging these AI-driven methods, haptic systems achieve higher levels of perception, prediction, and control, significantly enhancing the realism, safety, and adaptability of human–machine interaction in medical and robotic contexts.

2.7.1   Signal Processing and Classification

Raw force and tactile sensor data require preprocessing before AI inference. Bandpass filtering removes noise outside the physiologically relevant range (0.5–800 Hz for vibrotactile signals); normalization corrects for sensor drift; sliding-window segmentation creates fixed-length feature vectors suitable for neural network input. One-dimensional CNNs

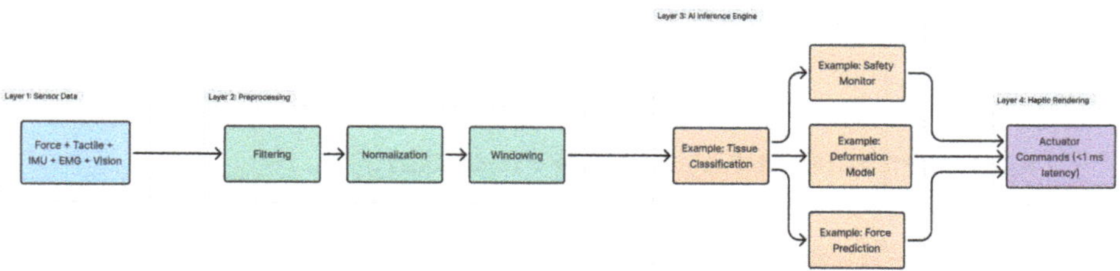

Fig. 2.5 AI pipeline for haptic data processing

Table 2.6 Tasks and applications of AI algorithms for haptic data processing

Algorithm	Task	Input	Haptic application
1D CNN	Signal classification	Force time series	Tissue type recognition
LSTM	Sequence prediction	Sensor streams	Predictive force rendering
Transformer	Multi-modal fusion	Force + vision	Context-aware haptic cues
Gaussian process	Uncertainty estimation	Sparse force samples	Safe robot impedance control
Reinforcement learning	Control optimization	State-action space	Adaptive haptic rendering
Bayesian neural net	Probabilistic output	Sensor + model	Confidence-aware feedback
Physics-informed NN	Deformation modelling	FEM + data	Real-time tissue simulation

applied to force time series achieve tissue classification accuracies above 95% for distinguishing healthy parenchyma, fibrous tissue, and tumour regions in ex vivo experiments [10]. Multi-modal fusion, combining concurrent force, vision, EMG, and IMU streams substantially improves classification accuracy. Transformer encoders applied to tokenized multi-modal sensor sequences learn cross-modal attention patterns, identifying, for example, that a visual cue of tissue blanching combined with elevated force corresponds to vascular compression even before force thresholds are exceeded [6].

2.7.2 Predictive Haptic Rendering

Teleoperation latency, the round-trip communication delay between surgeon and robot, is the fundamental barrier to realistic remote haptic feedback. Even 10 ms delays introduce perceptible instability in force-feedback loops. LSTM and Transformer sequence models trained on recorded haptic interactions learn to predict the force that the remote environment will exert 20–50 ms into the future, enabling the local haptic controller to render these predicted forces immediately, masking the true network delay [5, 10]. Prediction accuracy degrades for abrupt contacts and tool slippage events, motivating hybrid approaches that switch between predictive and passivity-based control depending on event confidence.

2.7.3 Reinforcement Learning for Adaptive Control

Reinforcement learning agents trained in simulation can acquire sophisticated haptic interaction policies, learning, for instance, to adjust grasping force in response to tissue deformation feedback so that force is always just sufficient to hold a suture without tearing tissue [14]. Sim-to-real transfer, the challenge of deploying simulation-trained RL agents on real robotic hardware with a different dynamics model is addressed through domain randomization (varying simulated material properties over a wide range during training) and real-world fine-tuning on limited hardware interaction data. Safety-constrained RL frameworks enforce force limits as hard constraints, ensuring compliance with the maximum allowable tissue contact forces specified during device design.

2.7.4 Generative Models for Haptic Simulation

Training data scarcity is a universal challenge in medical haptics; recording haptic interactions with real tissue requires expensive ex vivo or in vivo experimental setups. Generative adversarial networks (GANs) and diffusion models can synthesize realistic haptic signal trajectories conditioned on tissue type, surgical task, and force magnitude labels [10, 15]. Physics-informed neural networks [11] constrain generative models with the governing equations of tissue mechanics, ensuring that synthetic haptic data respects physical plausibility. These approaches have been shown to augment small real-tissue datasets by an order of magnitude, improving downstream tissue classifier accuracy by 8–15% points.

2.8 Summary

The chapter summarizes the foundational aspects of artificial intelligence (AI) and haptic systems relevant to healthcare. It highlights that AI comprises machine learning, deep learning, and symbolic reasoning, with machine learning approaches classified by the nature of supervision—supervised, unsupervised, and reinforcement learning. In medical contexts, convolutional neural networks (CNNs) are adept at identifying spatial patterns in images, while models like LSTMs and Transformers are designed to handle temporal and sequential information in clinical data. Federated and self-supervised learning are crucial for overcoming challenges related to limited data and privacy. On the haptic side, systems consist of actuators (for force, vibration, and temperature feedback) and diverse sensors (force/torque, tactile arrays, IMU, EMG), operating in a high-frequency rendering loop. Medical haptic hardware must meet strict requirements of stability, back drivability, and extremely low latency, and wearable devices enable broader clinical use despite facing design challenges. AI algorithms process haptic data for tissue perception, predictive and generative rendering, and adaptive control; advanced models help mitigate network delays and address the shortage of annotated training data in medical applications, ensuring responsive and intelligent tactile feedback for healthcare interventions.

References

1. LeCun, Y., Bengio, Y., & Hinton, G. (2015). Deep learning. *Nature, 521*(7553), 436–444.
2. Goodfellow, I., Bengio, Y., Courville, A., & Bengio, Y. (2016). *Deep learning* (pp. 1–800). MIT Press.
3. Litjens, G., Kooi, T., Bejnordi, B. E., Setio, A. A. A., Ciompi, F., Ghafoorian, M., et al. (2017). A survey on deep learning in medical image analysis. *Medical Image Analysis, 42*, 60–88.
4. Ronneberger, O., Fischer, P., & Brox, T. (2015, October). U-net: Convolutional networks for biomedical image segmentation. In *International conference on medical image computing and computer-assisted intervention* (pp. 234–241). Springer.
5. Hochreiter, S., & Schmidhuber, J. (1997). Long short-term memory. *Neural Computation, 9*(8), 1735–1780.
6. Vaswani, A., Shazeer, N., Parmar, N., Uszkoreit, J., Jones, L., Gomez, A. N., et al. (2017). Attention is all you need. *Advances in Neural Information Processing Systems, 30*.
7. Zhou, Q., Chen, Z. H., Cao, Y. H., & Peng, S. (2021). Clinical impact and quality of randomized controlled trials involving interventions evaluating artificial intelligence prediction tools: A systematic review. *npj Digital Medicine, 4*(1), 154.
8. Johansson, R. S., & Flanagan, J. R. (2009). Coding and use of tactile signals from the fingertips in object manipulation tasks. *Nature Reviews Neuroscience, 10*(5), 345–359.
9. Okamura, A. M. (2009). Haptic feedback in robot-assisted minimally invasive surgery. *Current Opinion in Urology, 19*(1), 102–107.
10. Laycock, S. D., & Day, A. M. (2007, March). A survey of haptic rendering techniques. *Computer Graphics Forum, 26*(1), 50–65.
11. Raissi, M., Perdikaris, P., & Karniadakis, G. E. (2019). Physics-informed neural networks: A deep learning framework for solving forward and inverse problems involving nonlinear partial differential equations. *Journal of Computational Physics, 378*, 686–707.
12. Pacchierotti, C., Sinclair, S., Solazzi, M., Frisoli, A., Hayward, V., & Prattichizzo, D. (2017). Wearable haptic systems for the fingertip and the hand: Taxonomy, review, and perspectives. *IEEE Transactions on Haptics, 10*(4), 580–600.
13. Shanmugam, M., Venusamy, K., Subin, S., Srivatsan, S., & Kumar, N. (2023, March). A comprehensive review of haptic gloves: Advances, challenges, and future directions. In *2023 Second International Conference on Electronics and Renewable Systems (ICEARS)* (pp. 227–233). IEEE.
14. Sutton, R. S., & Barto, A. G. (1998). *Reinforcement learning: An introduction* (pp. 9–11). MIT Press.
15. Esteva, A., Kuprel, B., Novoa, R. A., Ko, J., Swetter, S. M., Blau, H. M., & Thrun, S. (2017). Dermatologist-level classification of skin cancer with deep neural networks. *Nature, 542*(7639), 115–118.

AI-Driven Haptic Technologies and System Architecture

3

This chapter bridges the theoretical foundations established in Chap. 2 with the engineering realities of deploying AI-driven haptic systems in clinical environments. It systematically examines how intelligence is embedded in haptic interfaces, how AI and haptic hardware and software are integrated into coherent system architectures, and how real-time data processing pipelines achieve the sub-millisecond timing requirements of safe haptic interaction. The chapter then explores machine learning strategies for adaptive haptic responses, the edge-cloud computing continuum that supports healthcare AI devices, and the principles governing human–machine interaction in robotic surgical platforms. It concludes by synthesizing these threads into a set of evidence-based design principles for AI-enabled haptic medical systems including regulatory, safety, and usability considerations essential for clinical translation.

This chapter aims to provide a comprehensive understanding of intelligent haptic interfaces, ranging from rule-based systems to fully autonomous AI-driven solutions. It explores the integration of hardware and software layers for AI-haptic medical devices, emphasizing the importance of real-time data processing requirements and the technologies that address these demands in clinical haptic environments. Learners will evaluate machine learning approaches—including online reinforcement learning, meta-learning, and continual learning—for personalizing adaptive haptic responses. The chapter also analyses the trade-offs between edge and cloud computing in healthcare AI deployments, outlining hybrid architectures. Principles of human–machine interaction in robotic surgical systems are discussed, focusing on shared autonomy and safety-critical design. Finally, the chapter guides the application of structured design principles—such as safety, transparency, interoperability, and validation—to the development of AI-enabled haptic systems.

R. Thanki, *AI Role in Haptic Healthcare*, Synthesis Lectures on Biomedical Engineering, https://doi.org/10.1007/978-3-032-24907-4_3

3.1   Intelligent Haptic Interfaces

An intelligent haptic interface is a human–machine interaction system in which artificial intelligence augments, mediates, or generates the tactile communication channel between the user and the physical or virtual environment. The adjective 'intelligent' distinguishes these systems from classical haptic devices which execute deterministic, pre-programmed force profiles by their capacity to perceive context, learn from experience, and adapt their behaviour in response to patient variability, procedural state, and clinician performance [1, 2].

3.1.1   From Rule-Based to Autonomous Haptic Systems

The evolution of haptic interface intelligence can be mapped along a continuum from purely mechanical passive devices to fully autonomous systems capable of self-optimizing their interaction strategies [2]. Early robotic surgical tools implemented simple threshold-based haptic alerts: if measured contact force exceeded a pre-set limit, an audio tone or resistive force was triggered. While useful, these systems were brittle, unable to account for the wide inter-patient variability in tissue stiffness, surgical task context, or fatigue-induced changes in clinician motor control.

Supervised learning-based interfaces introduced the ability to classify tissue type in real time, enabling force profile modulation based on inferred tissue identity, applying greater caution near vessels and nerves than in fatty tissue. Adaptive AI interfaces using online reinforcement learning go further, updating their interaction policy continuously during a surgical procedure to personalize haptic responses to the individual patient's biomechanics and the specific surgeon's preference profile. Table 3.1 presents a systematic taxonomy of intelligent haptic interface classes.

Figure 3.1 depicts the architecture of an intelligent haptic interface system, highlighting the dynamic exchange of information between the clinician, the haptic device, an integrated sensor suite, an AI intelligence engine, and both physical and virtual environments. This bidirectional flow enables the system to interpret sensor data, classify and predict clinical scenarios, and provide actionable feedback to the clinician, all facilitated by the AI engine and its real-time connection to the environment and digital twin simulations.

3.1.2   Explainability in Intelligence Haptic Feedback

A critical but often overlooked dimension of intelligent haptic interfaces is explainability, the ability of the system to communicate the rationale behind AI-generated haptic cues to the clinician in real time. Without explainability, surgeons are presented with haptic signals whose origin is opaque, making it difficult to calibrate trust or detect system errors

Table 3.1 Taxonomy of intelligent haptic interface classes

Interface class	Intelligence layer	Key AI capability	Clinical application
Passive haptic	None (mechanical)	N/A	Basic surgical training rigs
Semi-active	Rule-based controller	Threshold alerting	Early robotic tool force limits
Supervised-AI haptic	Pre-trained classifier	Tissue-type detection	Robotic-assisted dissection
Adaptive AI haptic	Online RL/Bayesian	Personalized force tuning	Patient-specific rehabilitation
Predictive haptic	LSTM/Transformer	Latency-compensated rendering	Teleoperated remote surgery
Autonomous haptic	Multi-agent AI	Self-optimizing interaction	Autonomous suturing robots
Explainable haptic	XAI + haptic encoding	Interpretable surgical cues	AI-guided trainee feedback

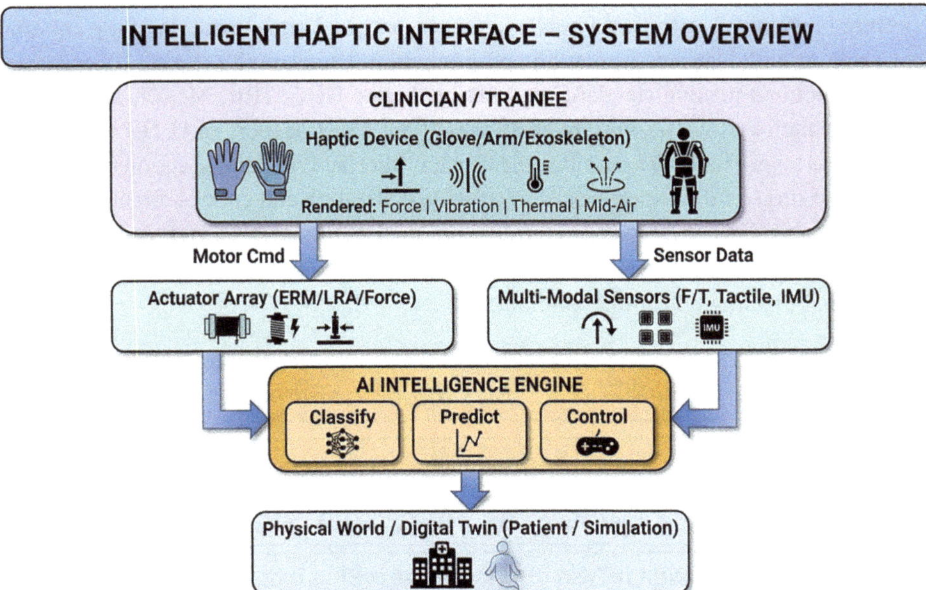

Fig. 3.1 Overview of intelligent haptic interface system

[3]. Explainable haptic systems encode the AI's confidence directly into the haptic modality: high-confidence tissue danger alerts may be rendered as sharp force impulses, while low-confidence advisory cues are conveyed as gentle vibrotactile patterns. Gradient-weighted activation maps (Grad-CAM) applied to the concurrent video stream can highlight the spatial tissue region responsible for a haptic warning, integrating visual and tactile explanatory channels [4].

3.2   Integration of AI with Haptic Hardware and Software

The integration of AI into a haptic system is not simply the addition of a machine learning model to an existing device. It requires holistic re-architecture of the system across hardware, firmware, middleware, and application layers, each layer imposing constraints on the others that must be resolved through careful systems engineering [2, 5].

Figure 3.2 illustrates the integration stack for AI-haptic medical systems, structured in seven distinct layers from the hardware up to the clinical interface. At the foundation (Layer 1), hardware components such as sensors, actuators, and FPGA controllers capture physical interactions and execute precise control. Layer 2 comprises the real-time operating system (like Xenomai or QNX), which manages high-frequency loops (typically 1 kHz) crucial for deterministic force rendering and safety-critical operations. Middleware (Layer 3, e.g. ROS 2 or DDS) facilitates robust message exchange between system components, ensuring seamless communication and synchronization.

AI inference (Layer 4) utilizes platforms such as TensorRT or ONNX, enabling rapid tissue classification with sub-millisecond latency. Above this, the digital twin layer (Layer 5, powered by Unity/Unreal and PhysX) maintains a virtual representation of the environment, supporting advanced simulation and prediction. Connectivity (Layer 6) integrates healthcare communication standards and protocols like HL7 FHIR, MQTT, and modern wireless technology (5G/Wi-Fi 6) to enable real-time data transport and EHR integration. The topmost layer (Layer 7) provides the clinical interface, including augmented reality overlays and surgeon user interfaces, delivering visualization and control directly to medical professionals. Data flows upward through the stack for processing and feedback, while control commands flow downward to actuators, creating a tightly integrated system for real-time, intelligent medical intervention.

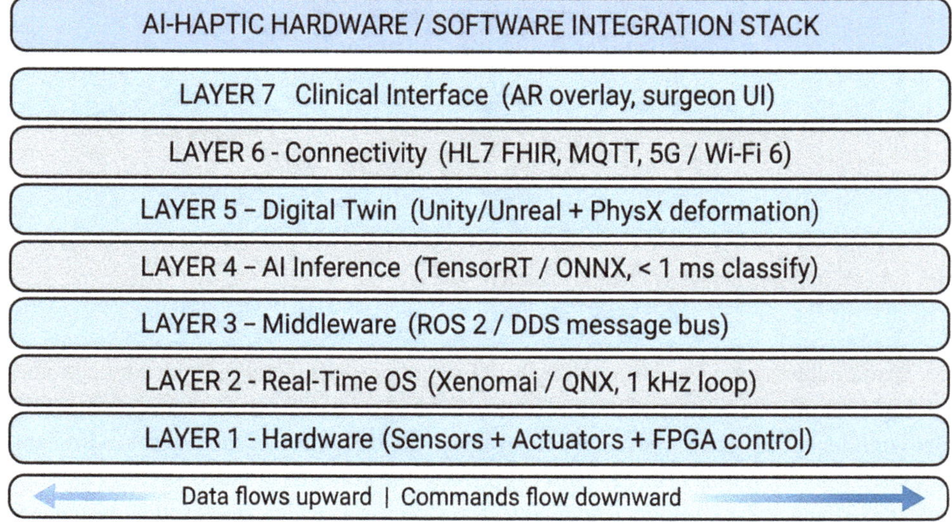

Fig. 3.2 Layered software integration stack for AI-haptic medical systems

Table 3.2 provides a structured overview of the software integration stack essential for AI-enhanced haptic systems. The table is organized by layers, each representing a foundational aspect of the overall system architecture. For each layer, the table lists the key components and the prevailing standards or technologies used and describes the specific role that layer plays within the AI-haptic system. By breaking down the AI-haptic system into these layers, Table 3.2 clarifies how hardware choices and software frameworks work together to meet the stringent demands of real-time, intelligent haptic feedback in clinical and research applications. This layered approach also facilitates modular development and easier integration of advanced AI components within robust and reliable haptic platforms.

3.2.1 Hardware–Software Co-design

The 1 kHz haptic rendering loop places hard real-time requirements on the entire signal path from sensor to actuator. AI inference must complete within the time budget of a single rendering cycle approximately 0.5–1 ms. Standard AI inference frameworks (TensorFlow, PyTorch) are not designed for deterministic real-time execution; they introduce variable garbage collection pauses and memory allocation delays incompatible with haptic timing requirements. TensorRT (NVIDIA) and ONNX Runtime address this by compiling neural network graphs into optimized hardware-specific kernels with deterministic execution profiles. For edge deployments on ARM-based systems, quantization to INT8 precision reduces both inference latency and memory footprint while maintaining clinically acceptable classification accuracy.

The communication bus architecture between sensing and actuation subsystems critically affects system latency. EtherCAT (Ethernet for Control Automation Technology) has emerged as the standard industrial fieldbus for high-performance haptic systems, achieving cycle times of 250 μs with sub-microsecond synchronization jitter across distributed

Table 3.2 AI-haptic software integration stack

Layer	Component	Standard/Technology	Role in AI-haptic system
Hardware	Actuators + sensors	EtherCAT, CAN bus	Physical interaction and measurement
Real-time OS	Haptic control loop	Xenomai, QNX, RTAI	1 kHz deterministic rendering
Middleware	ROS 2/DDS	ROS 2 Humble, Fast-DDS	Sensor-AI-actuator messaging
AI inference	Neural network runtime	TensorRT, ONNX Runtime	<1 ms tissue classification
Digital twin	Virtual environment model	Unity/Unreal + PhysX	Simulation and prediction
Clinical interface	Surgeon UI/AR overlay	OpenXR, DICOM RT	Visualization and control
Connectivity	Data transport	HL7 FHIR, MQTT, 5G	EHR integration and telemetry

nodes [5]. This determinism is essential when AI inference outputs must be translated into actuator commands without introducing perceptible haptic delay.

3.2.2 Regulatory Considerations in System Integration

From a regulatory perspective, the integration of AI into haptic medical devices introduces a system boundary challenge: the AI model constitutes a SaMD component subject to EU MDR 2017/745 classification and a software lifecycle governed by IEC 62304. Changes to the AI model including retraining new data or hyperparameter adjustment may constitute a modification to the medical device requiring regulatory re-evaluation [3, 6]. Predetermined change control plans (PCCPs) must be submitted to regulatory bodies before deployment, specifying the allowable boundary of AI model updates and the performance monitoring criteria that trigger re-validation. Audit trails capturing all AI model versions, inference inputs, and outputs must be maintained for post-market surveillance obligations.

3.3 Integration of AI with Haptic Hardware and Software

Real-time data processing in AI-haptic systems must satisfy two simultaneous and partially conflicting requirements: determinism (every computational deadline must be met, every time, without exception) and intelligence (the system must execute sophisticated AI inference to generate contextually appropriate haptic feedback) [2]. These requirements conflict because AI inference, particularly for large neural networks, involves variable computational workloads that are difficult to bound tightly. The engineering solution is a time-hierarchical processing architecture in which different processing tasks operate at different loop rates matched to their computational complexity and timing criticality. Figure 3.3 illustrates the architecture of a real-time data processing pipeline for advanced haptic feedback systems, such as those used in surgical robotics. At the top, multiple sensor streams—such as force and torque sensors, tactile arrays, inertial measurement units (IMUs), electromyography (EMG), and RGB-depth camera— continuously gather data about tool-tissue interactions and the environment. These diverse sensor modalities each operate with different sampling rates and have their own latency and noise characteristics.

The collected sensor data flows into the AI inference layers, where machine learning models, particularly deep learning fusion architectures like Transformer encoders, process and integrate multi-modal information. These models learn to dynamically prioritize the most relevant sensor signals depending on the context (e.g. focusing on tactile signals during suture placement, or force and vision for tissue retraction). Temporal alignment, achieved through hardware timestamp synchronization, ensures that all sensor data corresponds to the same physical moment for accurate analysis. Below the AI layers sits the haptic rendering engine, which interprets the fused sensor information and generates

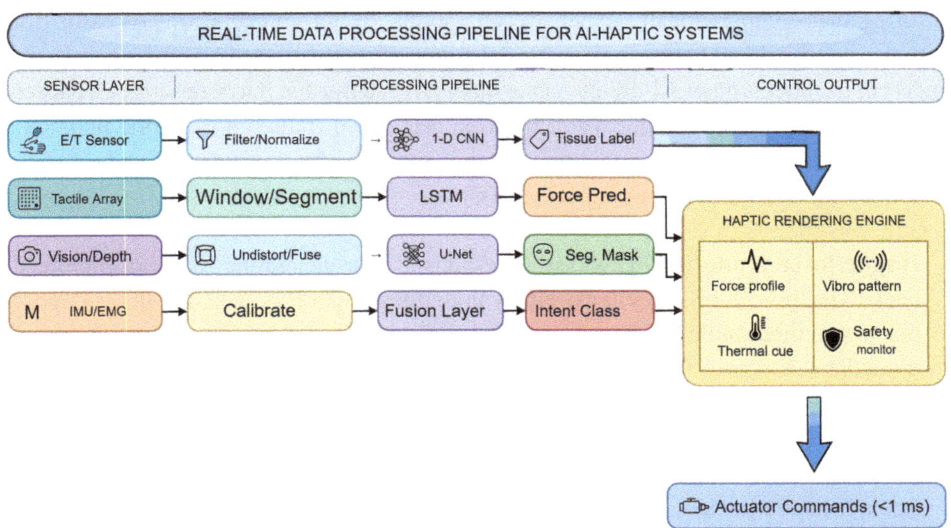

Fig. 3.3 Real-time AI-haptic data processing pipeline

commands for the actuators. The engine produces various feedback modalities, such as force profiles, vibration patterns, thermal cues, and safety monitoring signals. These outputs must be delivered to the actuators with extremely low latency—less than 1 ms—to ensure that the surgeon receives immediate, realistic tactile feedback.

The pipeline also incorporates real-time safety monitoring, which runs parallel to haptic rendering. This subsystem continuously checks incoming sensor readings and AI outputs against predefined safety thresholds. If anomalies are detected, such as unexpected tool behaviour or sensor failure, the system can trigger graduated safety responses, including haptic warnings, force limitation, or even halting actuator movement until clinical assessment is performed. In summary, Fig. 3.3 depicts how multi-modal sensor inputs are synchronized, analysed by AI inference layers, and translated by the haptic rendering engine into actuator commands with stringent timing requirements, all while maintaining continuous safety monitoring to protect both patient and operator.

3.3.1   Time-Hierarchical Processing Architecture

At the highest priority, the haptic force rendering loop executes at 1–2 kHz on a dedicated real-time processor or FPGA. This loop reads force/torque sensors, applies the current haptic rendering model (which may be a pre-computed lookup table, an analytic impedance model, or a lightweight neural network), and commands actuators all within 500 μs. AI tissue classification, operating at 50–200 Hz on a separate processor, asynchronously updates the haptic rendering parameters that the 1 kHz loop uses. Digital twin synchronization and cloud telemetry operate at even lower rates (10–30 Hz and 1 Hz, respectively), ensuring that computationally expensive operations do not compete for processor time with the safety-critical haptic loop. Table 3.3 summarizes the critical processing tasks that underpin the operation of AI-driven haptic medical systems. Each row describes a particular task, specifying how frequently it must be performed (required rate), the maximum allowable delay for completion (latency budget), and the technological solution best suited for achieving these demanding requirements.

- **Haptic force rendering:** This task is responsible for generating realistic force feedback to the user. It operates at extremely high rates (1–2 kHz), meaning it must update one to two thousand times per second. The latency budget is less than 0.5 ms, requiring immediate response. To meet these requirements, specialized hardware such as FPGAs (Field Programmable Gate Arrays) or real-time operating systems (RTOS) running on multi-core ARM processors are used.
- **Tactile texture rendering:** This involves creating the sensation of surface textures through haptic devices, running at 500–1000 Hz with a latency budget of less than 1 ms. GPU-accelerated signal synthesis is employed here, as graphics processing units (GPUs) are efficient at handling such high-speed signal generation.
- **Tissue classification (AI):** Using artificial intelligence, the system rapidly identifies different types of tissue. This process happens at 50–200 Hz and must finish within 5 ms. Edge GPUs using platforms like TensorRT (with INT8 precision) are used to achieve the necessary speed.
- **Force prediction (LSTM):** Long Short-Term Memory (LSTM) neural networks predict forces based on sensor inputs, operating at 100 Hz with a latency budget of less than 10 ms. ONNX Runtime on edge CPUs is the preferred technology, balancing speed, and computational power.
- **Image-guided haptic update:** Updates to haptic feedback guided by real-time imaging data occur at 25–60 Hz and must complete in less than 16 ms. This task leverages GPU inference and high-speed USB3 vision interfaces for rapid processing.
- **Digital twin sync:** Synchronization with a digital twin (a virtual model of the physical environment) occurs at 10–30 Hz, with a latency budget under 33 ms. Technologies such as ROS 2 DDS (a middleware for robotic systems) and PhysX GPU (for physics simulation) are used.

Table 3.3 Real-time processing requirements for AI-haptic systems

Processing task	Required rate	Latency budget	Technology solution
Haptic force rendering	1–2 kHz	<0.5 ms	FPGA/RTOS on multi-core ARM
Tactile texture rendering	500–1000 Hz	<1 ms	GPU-accelerated signal synthesis
Tissue classification (AI)	50–200 Hz	<5 ms	TensorRT INT8 on edge GPU
Force prediction (LSTM)	100 Hz	<10 ms	ONNX Runtime on edge CPU
Image-guided haptic update	25–60 Hz	<16 ms	GPU inference + USB3 vision
Digital twin sync	10–30 Hz	<33 ms	ROS 2 DDS + PhysX GPU
Telemetry to cloud/EHR	0.1–1 Hz	<1 s	MQTT over 5G or Wi-Fi 6

- **Telemetry to cloud/EHR:** Transmission of system data to the cloud or electronic health records happens at a slower rate (0.1–1 Hz), with a latency budget of less than 1 s. Communication is facilitated by MQTT protocol over high-speed wireless networks like 5G or Wi-Fi 6.

In summary, Table 3.3 demonstrates how different system components operate at tailored rates and with strict timing constraints, supported by specific hardware and software platforms. This time-hierarchical architecture ensures that safety-critical and high-speed feedback tasks are prioritized, while computationally intensive or less urgent tasks are handled at lower frequencies, maintaining both determinism and intelligent responsiveness in AI-haptic medical systems.

3.3.2   Multi-Modal Sensor Fusion

Rich haptic feedback generation requires integrating information from multiple concurrent sensor streams: force/torque, tactile arrays, inertial measurement units (IMUs), electromyography (EMG), and RGB-depth vision. Each sensor modality has a different sampling rate, signal-to-noise ratio, and latency profile. Temporal alignment ensuring that samples from different sensors corresponding to the same physical moment are processed together requires hardware timestamp synchronization, typically achieved through hardware trigger signals distributed via EtherCAT or IEEE 1588 Precision Time Protocol [5]. Deep learning fusion architectures, particularly Transformer encoders applied to multimodal token sequences [7], learn cross-modal attention patterns that identify the most informative combination of sensor signals for each contextual state. For example, during suture placement, the model learns to weight tactile slip signals heavily while deprioritizing EMG, whereas during tissue retraction, force magnitude and vision-estimated tissue deformation are weighted more strongly. This dynamic attention-based weighting substantially outperforms static feature concatenation approaches in tissue classification and force prediction accuracy.

3.3.3   Safety Monitoring and Fault Detection

Real-time safety monitoring must operate in parallel with haptic rendering, continuously checking sensor readings and AI outputs against pre-validated safety envelopes. Anomaly detection models, typically autoencoders or one-class SVMs trained on nominal operating data, raise alerts when sensor patterns deviate from the expected distribution, potentially indicating sensor failure, unexpected anatomy, or loss of tool-tissue contact [2]. Upon alert, the system implements a graduated response: first, a haptic warning to the surgeon; if unacknowledged, a progressive force limit reduction; and finally, a hold-in-place command to the robotic actuators pending clinical assessment. This multi-level response hierarchy is specified in the device's hazard analysis and risk management file under ISO 14971.

3.4 Machine Learning for Adaptive Haptic Responses

A defining capability of AI-driven haptic systems over classical systems is adaptivity, the ability to modify haptic rendering behaviour in response to new information. Adaptation operates at multiple time scales: within a surgical procedure (intra-operative), across sessions with the same patient (inter-session), and across the patient population (population-level) [8, 9]. Each time scale demands different machine learning strategies.

3.4.1 Intra-Operative Adaptation via Reinforcement Learning

Online reinforcement learning enables a haptic system to update its interaction policy in real time during a procedure, adapting to the specific biomechanics of the individual patient's tissue. The system models the interaction as a Markov Decision Process: the state includes current force readings, tissue classification, tool position, and task progress; the action is the haptic rendering parameter set; and the reward combines tissue integrity metrics, task efficiency, and surgeon preference signals [8]. Policy gradient algorithms, particularly Proximal Policy Optimisation (PPO) and Soft Actor-Critic (SAC), are favoured for their sample efficiency and stable convergence in continuous action spaces. Safety-constrained RL is mandatory in clinical applications. Constrained Policy Optimisation (CPO) and Lagrangian RL methods enforce hard limits on contact force and insertion depth as inequality constraints in the policy optimization problem, ensuring that the RL agent never learns to violate safety boundaries even when doing so would yield higher reward [8].

Figure 3.4 illustrates how adaptive haptic responses are achieved through online machine learning, specifically reinforcement learning, within surgical procedures. This process is known as the 'ML Online Learning Loop' for haptic feedback. At its core, the system operates in episodes of interaction with the environment, which includes the patient's tissue and the surgical task. Each episode begins by capturing the current state (s) such as force readings, tissue type, tool position, and task progress. This state is processed by a policy (π), which determines the optimal action (a). In this context, the action is a specific haptic command that controls the feedback felt by the surgeon.

The action is then executed in the environment (the patient's tissue or anatomy), causing a change that leads to a new state (s'). The system then evaluates the outcome using a reward signal (r), which is a function of tissue integrity, task efficiency, and surgeon preferences. This reward guides the learning process, helping the system understand whether the action taken was beneficial or not. All these interactions are stored in a replay buffer, which accumulates experiences from multiple episodes. The policy is then updated using

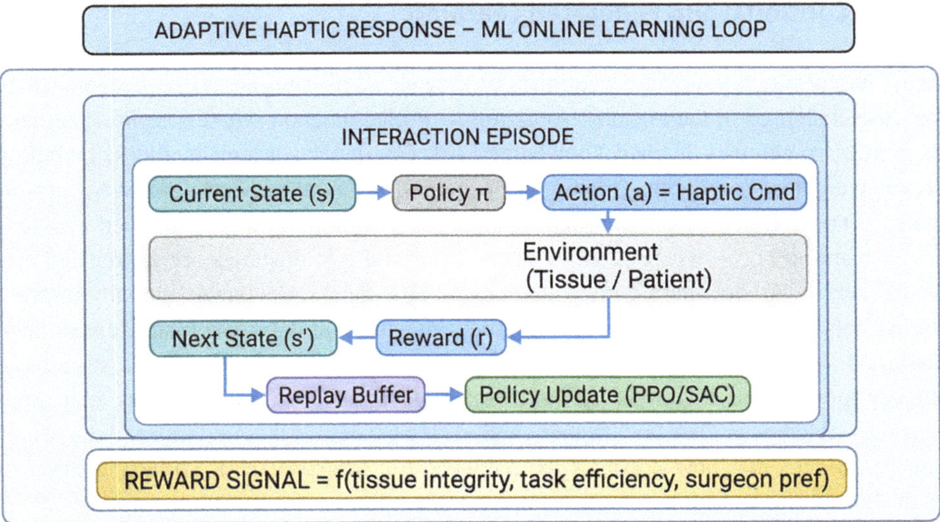

Fig. 3.4 Adaptive haptic response through online reinforcement learning

advanced reinforcement learning algorithms such as Proximal Policy Optimization (PPO) or Soft Actor-Critic (SAC). These updates enable the system to improve its decision-making over time, adapting the haptic feedback to the patient's unique tissue characteristics and the surgeon's preferences.

Importantly, this loop operates within safety-constrained boundaries. The system ensures that actions never violate safety limits, such as excessive force or depth, even if doing so might increase the reward. This is achieved through safety-constrained reinforcement learning methods, which enforce hard constraints during policy optimization. In summary, the diagram shows the continuous cycle of sensing, acting, learning, and updating that allows AI-driven haptic systems to personalize feedback in real time during surgery, while always maintaining patient safety.

3.4.2 Inter-Session Adaptation via Meta-Learning

Meta-learning or learning to learn trains a model on a distribution of tasks such that it can rapidly adapt to a new task with minimal data [9]. In the haptic context, Model-Agnostic Meta-Learning (MAML) pre-trains a haptic policy on data from many patients, learning initial model weights that are close to the optimal policy for any new patient and can be fine-tuned with just a few interactions. This is clinically valuable because comprehensive haptic data collection from a new patient before surgery is infeasible; the system must instead initialize effectively and adapt rapidly from the first few tool-tissue contacts of the procedure.

3.4.3 Continual and Federated Learning

As AI-haptic systems accumulate clinical experience across thousands of procedures, they face the challenge of catastrophic forgetting— a phenomenon where retraining on new data erases previously learned knowledge [10]. Continual learning methods, including elastic weight consolidation (EWC) and progressive neural networks, preserve performance on prior tasks while incorporating knowledge from new ones. Combined with federated learning [11]—where model updates from multiple hospitals are aggregated at a central server without sharing raw patient data these approaches enable globally improving AI-haptic systems that respect GDPR and institutional data governance constraints. Table 3.4 summarizes key machine learning algorithms used to make haptic systems in surgery more adaptive and personalized. Each algorithm is described by its adaptation type (how it learns or changes), trigger condition (what causes it to update), and the resulting haptic outcome (how it affects the feedback the surgeon feels). The explanation of each algorithm is as follows:

- **Online RL (PPO/SAC):** Uses reinforcement learning to update its policy in real time for each patient, creating a personalized profile for haptic feedback based on the patient's tissue and surgeon's preferences.
- **Bayesian Optimization:** Tune system parameters (like rendering gain) to optimize haptic feedback for the session, based on overall performance.
- **Gaussian Process Regression:** Updates the system when it is uncertain about its predictions, ensuring that force limits remain safe and conservative.
- **Meta-Learning (MAML):** Quickly adapts to new patients or tissue types using only a few examples, starting from a model trained on many previous cases.

Table 3.4 Machine learning algorithms for adaptive haptic responses

Algorithm	Adaptation type	Trigger condition	Haptic outcome
Online RL (PPO/SAC)	Policy update	Each patient encounter	Personalized impedance profile
Bayesian optimization	Hyperparameter tuning	Session-level performance	Optimal rendering gain
Gaussian process regression	Uncertainty-aware update	Low-confidence prediction	Conservative safe force limit
Meta-learning (MAML)	Few-shot adaptation	New tissue/patient type	Rapid profile initialization
Continual learning	Non-forgetting update	New clinical tasks added	Knowledge retention across tasks
Active learning	Query strategy	High-uncertainty samples	Efficient annotation requests
Transfer learning	Domain shift handling	New surgical procedure	Pre-trained feature reuse

- **Continual Learning:** Allows the system to learn new tasks without forgetting previous ones, so it keeps knowledge from earlier clinical experiences even as it adapts to new ones.
- **Active Learning:** Focuses annotation efforts on the most uncertain cases, improving efficiency by asking for expert input only when needed.
- **Transfer Learning:** Reuses features learned from previous procedures to adapt quickly to new types of surgeries, helping the system handle changes in domain or task.

In summary, these algorithms work together to make haptic systems smarter, safer, and more responsive to both patient and surgeon needs, while continuously learning and adapting in clinical environments.

3.5   Edge Computing and Cloud Support in Healthcare Devices

The deployment of AI in healthcare haptic systems raises a fundamental architectural question: where should computation reside? The answer determines system latency, data privacy exposure, regulatory complexity, and resilience to connectivity failures [12]. Three deployment patterns are relevant: pure edge computing (all inference on the device), pure cloud computing (interference in remote data centres), and hybrid edge-cloud architectures that distribute computation according to task criticality and data sensitivity.

3.5.1   Edge Computing for Safety-Critical Haptic Control

Safety-critical haptic control, the 1 kHz force rendering loop, real-time tissue classification, and safety monitoring must execute at the edge (on-device or within the operating theatre) to guarantee the sub-millisecond latency requirements [6]. Modern edge AI accelerators, including the NVIDIA Jetson Orin (275 TOPS), Google Coral TPU, and Intel Movidius VPU, provide sufficient computers for running quantized neural network inference at haptic rates on platforms small enough for integration into surgical robot consoles or wearable training systems. On-device processing also minimizes the exposure of sensitive patient biomechanical data to network transmission, directly supporting GDPR Article 25 (Data Protection by Design) compliance.

3.5.2   Cloud Computing for Population-Level Learning

Population-level model retraining, large-scale analytics, and the training of foundation models require compute resources that far exceed edge capabilities. Cloud platforms (AWS Health Lake, Microsoft Azure Health Data Services, Google Cloud Healthcare API) provide storage, compute, and HIPAA/GDPR-compliant infrastructure for aggregating de-identified haptic procedure data and retraining global AI models [3]. Model updates are then pushed back to edge devices via over-the-air (OTA) update mechanisms, subject to regulatory change control procedures. The cloud platform also hosts population monitoring dashboards that visualize procedure outcome metrics, AI model performance drift, and adverse event patterns providing the real-world evidence required for post-market clinical follow-up (PMCF) under EU MDR.

3.5.3 Hybrid Edge-Cloud Architecture

The recommended architecture for clinical AI-haptic deployments is a hybrid model that assigns each computational function to the tier best suited to its latency, privacy, and computation requirements [11, 12]. Haptic control and safety monitoring are pinned to the edge; medium-priority functions such as procedure logging and digital twin synchronization use local hospital servers; population learning and regulatory analytics reside in the cloud. Federated learning connects these tiers: local models are trained on edge data, and their gradient updates are aggregated in the cloud without raw data leaving the hospital network, satisfying both performance and privacy objectives. Table 3.5 and Fig. 3.5 compare the three deployment options across key attributes.

3.6   Robotics and Human–Machine Interaction

Robotic surgical systems are the primary deployment context for AI-driven haptic technologies in clinical practice. These systems mediate the surgeon's physical interaction with the patient through a complex sociotechnical layer comprising robotic kinematics, haptic rendering, visual feedback, and AI intelligence creating a human–machine interaction (HMI) environment qualitatively different from conventional surgery [13, 14].

Figure 3.6 illustrates the different layers of interaction between humans and machines in the context of AI-haptic robotic surgery. The diagram presents a continuum of shared autonomy, ranging from full manual control by the surgeon, progressing through AI-assisted modes, co-pilot arrangements, and culminating in supervised autonomy. At each stage along this continuum, the role of AI changes—from not being involved (full manual), to providing alerts and advisory feedback, assisting with force-limited actions, and ultimately enabling autonomous operation with human override capabilities.

The interaction layers also highlight the flow of information and control: awareness cues (such as explainable AI signals), haptic feedback, command inputs, and instrument actions (like tissue manipulation) are distributed across the continuum. This structure ensures that as the level of autonomy increases, AI systems take on more responsibility for monitoring, assisting, and managing safety, while still allowing the surgeon to intervene or override as needed. The design aligns with principles discussed in the surrounding text, such as safety-by-design and adaptive haptic information, supporting both patient and surgeon safety while optimizing cognitive workload and system transparency.

Table 3.5 Edge vs. cloud vs. hybrid computing for healthcare AI-haptic deployments

Attribute	Edge computing	Cloud computing	Hybrid approach
Latency	<1 ms (local)	50–200 ms	<5 ms critical/cloud analytics
Data privacy	High (on device)	Risk (data leaves device)	Federated—Raw data stays local
Computer power	Moderate (GPU/TPU)	Very high (HPC clusters)	Balance per task criticality
Model complexity	Small–medium (<100 M params)	Very large (LLM-scale)	Distilled edge + full cloud
Availability	Offline-capable	Internet required	Graceful offline degradation
Updates	Scheduled OTA	Real-time retraining	Federated gradient aggregation
Regulatory risk	Lower (GDPR local)	Higher (data transfer)	Risk-stratified architecture

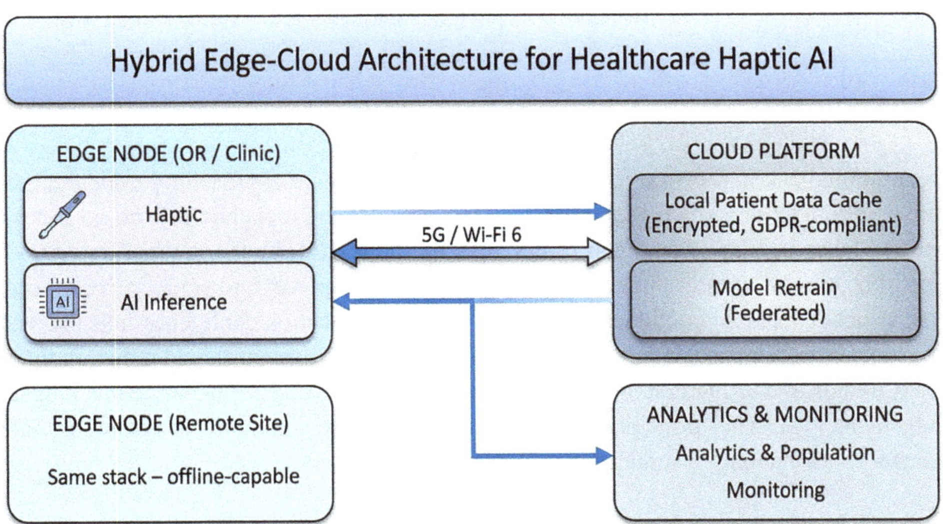

Fig. 3.5 Hybrid edge-cloud architecture for AI-haptic healthcare systems

3.6.1   Shared Autonomy in Surgical Robotics

The concept of shared autonomy describes a spectrum of human–robot collaboration in which control authority is dynamically distributed between the human surgeon and the robotic AI system based on task context, surgeon performance state, and system confidence [14]. At one extreme, the surgeon has full manual control and the robot acts as a precision instrument, faithfully scaling and filtering hand motions. At the other extreme, a supervised autonomous robot performs procedural steps independently, with the surgeon available to intervene. Between these poles, AI-haptic systems can implement

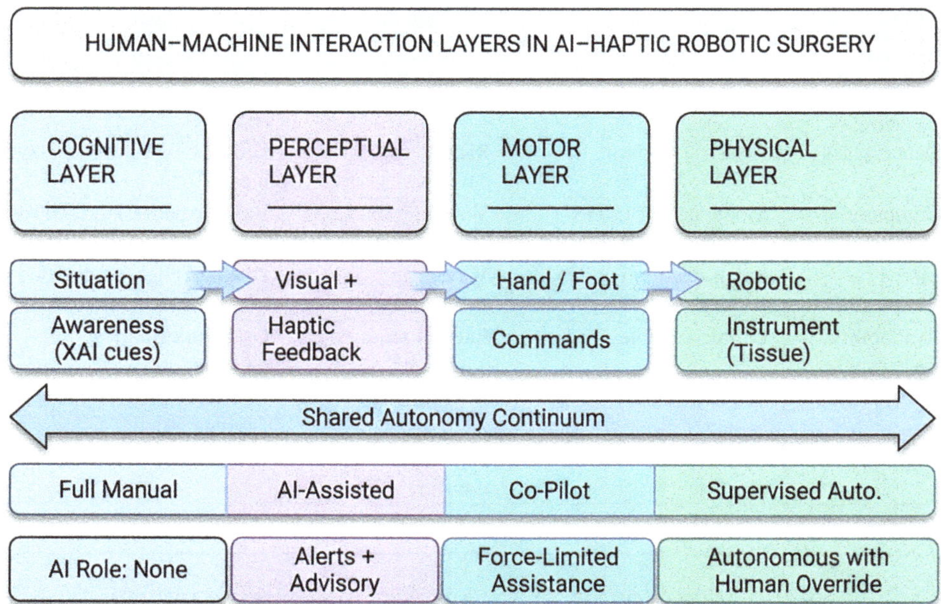

Fig. 3.6 Human–machine interaction layers in AI-haptic robotic surgery

force-limited assistance (the robot gently resists movements approaching critical structures), virtual fixtures (hard geometric constraints preventing tool entry into no-go zones), and guidance haptics (directional forces steering the tool along the optimal trajectory). The allocation of control authority must be dynamic, responsive to surgeon preference, task criticality, and AI confidence. When AI tissue classification confidence falls below a threshold indicating an ambiguous anatomical situation, the system should reduce autonomous authority and increase haptic advisory signals, deferring to the surgeon's clinical judgement [15]. This principle of confidence-contingent autonomy is central to safe human–robot teaming in surgical environments.

3.6.2   Physical Human–Robot Interaction Safety

Physical human–robot interaction (pHRI) safety in surgical robotics encompasses both patient safety (preventing inadvertent tissue damage by the robot) and surgeon safety (preventing injury from unexpected robot motion during teleoperation) [14]. ISO/TS 15066 specifies biomechanical pain and injury thresholds for collaborative robot–human contact forces, providing the quantitative limits that AI-haptic safety monitoring systems must enforce. Impedance control, which models the robot as a virtual spring-damper system and limits its force response to external contacts, is the dominant safety control paradigm for collaborative surgical robots. AI augments pHRI safety through predictive collision avoidance: recurrent neural networks trained on prior procedure data predict tool trajectories 100–500 ms into the future, enabling the robot to pro-actively impose force limits before a potentially unsafe contact occurs rather than reacting after it [10]. Anomaly detection models continuously monitor the consistency between intended and observed robot state, flagging deviations that may indicate external interference, patient movement, or mechanical fault.

3.6.3   Cognitive Load and Haptic Information Design

Surgeons operating robotic systems with rich AI-haptic feedback are simultaneously managing visual information, task planning, team communication, and haptic cues, a high cognitive load environment where poorly designed haptic signals can cause information overload and degrade performance [13]. Haptic information design principles derived from psychophysics and human factors research specify that haptic warnings should be discriminable from background interaction forces, spatially congruent with their anatomical source, and modality-appropriate: force cues for directional guidance, vibrotactile for texture and slip, and thermal for tissue state. Adaptive haptic priority queuing, an AI mechanism that ranks competing haptic alerts and presents only the most critical within each rendering cycle, prevents alert overload during complex multi-hazard scenarios.

3.7   Design Principles for AI-Enabled Haptic Systems

The design of AI-enabled haptic systems for clinical deployment requires reconciling the demands of biomedical engineering, AI development, regulatory compliance, and human-centred design. The following principles synthesize guidance from international standards, clinical evidence, and engineering best practice into an actionable framework for developers [3, 6]. Table 3.6 gives standards and metrics required to design any AI-Enabled Haptic Systems for healthcare.

3.7.1   Safety-by-Design

Safety must be designed in from the earliest architectural decisions, not added as a post-hoc layer. ISO 14971:2019 risk management mandates systematic hazard identification (FMEA, FTA) covering both hardware failures and AI model failures including out-of-distribution inputs, adversarial perturbations, and distributional shift after deployment [6]. Safety-relevant AI functions such as tissue classification used to enforce force limits, for example, must be implemented at Software Safety Integrity Level 2 or above (IEC 61508), requiring rigorous testing across the full input distribution including edge cases and failure modes.

Table 3.6 Design principles for AI-enabled haptic systems

Design principle	Standard/framework	Metric	Haptic system implication
Safety-by-design	IEC 62304, ISO 14971	FMEA severity score	Force limits as hard constraints
Transparency	ISO/IEC 42001 XAI	Explanation fidelity	Surgeon-legible haptic cues
Minimize cognitive load	ISO 9241-210 HCD	Task completion time	Haptic priority queuing
Redundancy and fail-safe	IEC 61508 SIL-2	MTBF, fault detection rate	Dual-channel force monitoring
Adaptability	GDPR Art. 25, HIPAA	Personalization accuracy	Per-patient force profile storage
Interoperability	HL7 FHIR R4, IHE	API conformance score	EHR-linked haptic parameter sets
Validation and V&V	ISO 13485, FDA 21 CFR 820	Clinical trial endpoints	Simulation-to-OR fidelity testing

3.7.2 Transparency and Explainability

ISO/IEC 42001 (AI Management Systems) and the EU AI Act both require that high-risk AI systems including those deployed in surgical and clinical decision support contexts provide meaningful explanations of their decisions to qualified users [3]. In the haptic domain, this means encoding AI confidence and rationale into the haptic signal itself: graduated force resistance proportional to classification confidence, vibrotactile patterns distinguishing 'vessel proximity' from 'nerve proximity' warnings, and concurrent visual overlays providing anatomical context for haptic cues. User studies measuring surgeon understanding of AI-generated haptic signals are a regulatory expectation in clinical evaluation protocols.

3.7.3 Interoperability and Standards Compliance

AI-haptic systems must interoperate with hospital information systems, electronic health records, and other medical devices. HL7 FHIR R4 provides the data exchange standard for patient-linked haptic procedure parameters and outcome data. DICOM extensions cover imaging-linked haptic simulation data. IHE profiles (Integrating the Healthcare Enterprise) specify implementation guidance for clinical workflow integration [5]. Adopting open standards from the outset rather than proprietary data formats substantially reduces integration costs, accelerates regulatory review, and enables multi-vendor interoperability.

3.7.4 Validation, Verification, and Clinical Evidence

Verification (does the system do what the design specification says?) and validation (does the system meet user needs in the intended clinical environment?) are both mandatory under ISO 13485:2016 and EU MDR [6]. For AI components, validation must demonstrate performance across the full intended patient population including demographic subgroups, anatomical variations, and procedural contexts. Simulation-based testing cannot substitute for clinical evidence: Class IIb and III AI-haptic systems require prospective clinical investigations with pre-specified primary endpoints, sample size calculations, and statistical analysis plans filed with the notified body before the study begins. Post-market clinical follow-up (PMCF) plans must specify how AI model performance will be monitored in real-world use and what triggers a corrective action or regulatory re-submission.

3.8 Summary

This chapter delves into the integration of AI-driven haptic technologies within clinical environments, focusing on system architecture, real-time data processing, and adaptive machine learning strategies. It explores the evolution of haptic interfaces from passive mechanical devices to fully autonomous systems capable of personalized responses through reinforcement learning, meta-learning, and continual learning. The chapter emphasizes the importance of explainability in haptic feedback, ensuring clinicians understand AI-generated cues, and discusses the layered integration of hardware and software for real-time, intelligent haptic systems. It also highlights the trade-offs between edge and cloud computing, advocating for a hybrid architecture to balance latency, privacy, and computational needs.

The chapter further examines human–machine interaction in robotic surgical systems, emphasizing shared autonomy, physical safety, and cognitive load management. It concludes with evidence-based design principles for AI-enabled haptic systems, including safety-by-design, transparency, adaptability, interoperability, and regulatory compliance. By synthesizing engineering, clinical, and regulatory considerations, the chapter provides a comprehensive framework for developing intelligent haptic systems that enhance surgical precision, safety, and usability in healthcare settings.

References

1. Okamura, A. M. (2009). Haptic feedback in robot-assisted minimally invasive surgery. *Current Opinion in Urology, 19*(1), 102–107.
2. Zhou, Q., Chen, Z. H., Cao, Y. H., & Peng, S. (2021). Clinical impact and quality of randomized controlled trials involving interventions evaluating artificial intelligence prediction tools: A systematic review. *npj Digital Medicine, 4*(1), 154.

3. World Health Organization. (2023). *Regulatory considerations on artificial intelligence for health*. World Health Organization.
4. Topol, E. J. (2019). High-performance medicine: The convergence of human and artificial intelligence. *Nature Medicine, 25*(1), 44–56.
5. Quigley, M., Conley, K., Gerkey, B., Faust, J., Foote, T., Leibs, J., et al. (2009, May). ROS: An open-source Robot Operating System. In *ICRA workshop on open source software* (Vol. 3, No. 3.2, p. 5).
6. International Organization for Standardization. (2022). *ISO 13485:2016/AMD 1:2022—Medical devices: Quality management systems*. ISO.
7. Vaswani, A., Shazeer, N., Parmar, N., Uszkoreit, J., Jones, L., Gomez, A. N., et al. (2017). Attention is all you need. *Advances in Neural Information Processing Systems, 30*.
8. Sutton, R. S., & Barto, A. G. (1998). *Reinforcement learning: An introduction* (pp. 9–11). MIT Press.
9. Finn, C., Abbeel, P., & Levine, S. (2017, July). Model-agnostic meta-learning for fast adaptation of deep networks. In *International conference on machine learning* (pp. 1126–1135). PMLR.
10. Li, Z., & Hoiem, D. (2018). Learning without forgetting. *IEEE Transactions on Pattern Analysis and Machine Intelligence, 40*(12), 2935–2947. https://doi.org/10.1109/TPAMI.2017.2773081
11. McMahan, B., Moore, E., Ramage, D., Hampson, S., & y Arcas, B. A. (2017, April). Communication-efficient learning of deep networks from decentralized data. In *Artificial intelligence and statistics* (pp. 1273–1282). PMLR.
12. Shi, W., Cao, J., Zhang, Q., Li, Y., & Xu, L. (2016). Edge computing: Vision and challenges. *IEEE Internet of Things Journal, 3*(5), 637–646.
13. Riek, L. D. (2017). Healthcare robotics. *Communications of the ACM, 60*(11), 68–78.
14. Haddadin, S., & Croft, E. (2016). Physical human–robot interaction. In *Springer handbook of robotics* (pp. 1835–1874). Springer.
15. Zemmar, A., Lozano, A. M., & Nelson, B. J. (2020). The rise of robots in surgical environments during COVID-19. *Nature Machine Intelligence, 2*(10), 566–572.

Applications of AI-Powered Haptic Technology in Healthcare

4

This chapter translates the architectural and algorithmic foundations of Chaps. 2 and 3 into the diverse clinical applications where AI-powered haptic technology is demonstrating measurable impact. The seven application domains examined—robotic surgery, medical simulation, rehabilitation, smart prosthetics, telemedicine, pain management, and a dedicated case study section—together form the broadest clinical deployment landscape for AI-haptic systems in contemporary healthcare. The chapter integrates real-world use cases from industry practice, including a detailed examination of haptic communication in healthcare covering remote consultation, rehabilitation guidance, clinical alerting, surgical navigation, and assistive technologies for visually impaired patients. Each section presents the engineering underpinnings, clinical evidence base, AI integration architecture, and outstanding challenges for its respective domain.

The learning objectives of this chapter are as follows: to describe how AI-haptic integration restores and enhances tactile feedback in robotic minimally invasive surgery, to explain the architecture and clinical value of AI-driven haptic medical simulation and training systems, to evaluate AI-haptic rehabilitation platforms for neurological and musculoskeletal recovery supported by clinical evidence, to analys AI-enabled sensory feedback mechanisms in smart prosthetics and brain–computer interfaces, to assess telemedicine haptic architectures for remote palpation, tele-surgery, and remote physiotherapy, to describe AI-haptic modalities as applied in pain management, sensory therapy, and VR analgesia, and to critically evaluate real-world use cases in haptic communication for healthcare, including IoMT-based predictive models.

R. Thanki, *AI Role in Haptic Healthcare*, Synthesis Lectures on Biomedical Engineering, https://doi.org/10.1007/978-3-032-24907-4_4

4.1   Robotic Surgery with Haptic Feedback

Robotic minimally invasive surgery (RMIS) represents the most clinically mature deployment context for AI-haptic integration. Current robotic surgical platforms led by Intuitive Surgical's da Vinci family have accumulated over ten million procedures globally, demonstrating benefits including reduced intraoperative blood loss, faster patient recovery, and shorter hospital stays. Yet these platforms have long been criticized for eliminating tactile feedback: the electromechanical transmission of force information from instruments to surgeon is either absent or severely attenuated, creating the 'haptic deficit' that compromises tissue handling safety and increases the cognitive demand on the operating surgeon [1].

Figure 4.1 visually represents how information travels within an AI-enabled robotic surgery system, highlighting the two-way communication between the surgeon and the surgical robot. The diagram begins with the surgeon console, where the surgeon controls robotic instruments. Signals from the console are sent to the robotic platform, which physically manipulates the surgical tools.

Integrated into the robotic platform is a sensor suite that captures raw data, including force and vibration feedback (haptic feedback), during tissue interaction. This sensor data is continuously fed to the AI inference engine, which analyses it in real time. The AI engine performs critical functions such as tissue classification, predictive force rendering, and safety monitoring. For example, it can distinguish between different types of tissue (like vessel, nerve, or tumour margin) and predict the amount of force needed to safely manipulate them.

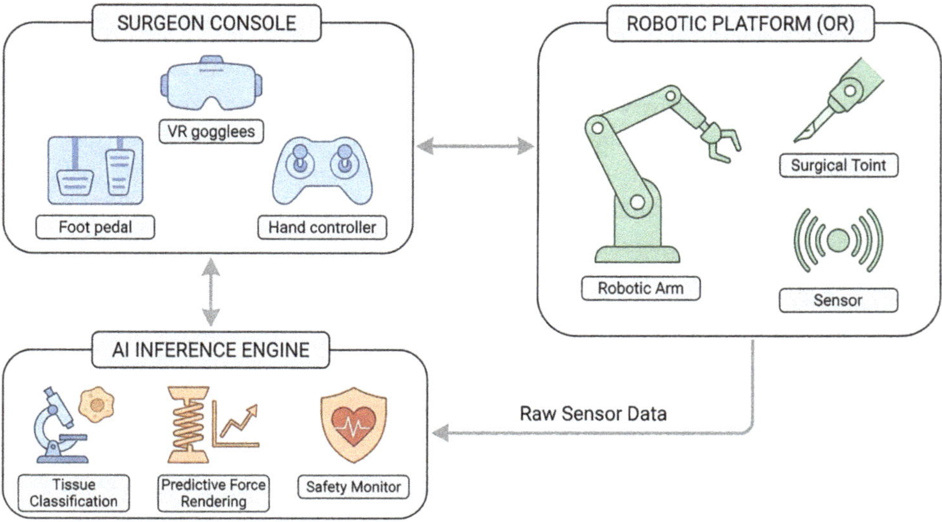

Fig. 4.1 Information flow on AI-haptic robotic surgery

Table 4.1 provides an overview of several advanced robotic surgical platforms, highlighting their developers, haptic feedback modalities, and how artificial intelligence (AI) is integrated into their clinical applications.

- Da Vinci Xi by Intuitive Surgical offers limited force scaling, mainly used for laparoscopic and thoracic procedures. AI add-ons can alert surgeons about tissue types and risks.
- Hugo RAS from Medtronic features both vibrotactile and force feedback, supporting fields like urology and gynaecology. AI helps control surgical instruments more precisely.
- SPORT Surgical by Titan Medical provides six degrees of freedom (6-DOF) force feedback for single-incision procedures. AI is used to predict the amount of force needed during operations.
- Versius developed by CMR Surgical uses kinaesthetic resistance to enhance general surgery. It also applies real-time AI analytics to monitor and improve surgical performance.
- Raven II (research) from the University of Washington is an open-source platform offering full force feedback. It uses reinforcement learning (RL) for haptic control, making it adaptable for various research applications.
- MAESTRO (research) by BioRobotics Lab incorporates multi-modal tactile feedback, primarily for microsurgery. AI is employed for tissue classification, helping surgeons distinguish between different tissue types.
- Symani Surgical from MMI includes tremor filtering and force feedback, designed for microsurgical tasks involving structures less than 3 mm in size. AI scales motion mapping, providing precision in delicate procedures.

Table 4.1 Robotic surgical platforms

Platform	Developer	Haptic modality	Clinical application and AI integration
da Vinci Xi [2]	Intuitive Surgical	Force scaling (limited)	Laparoscopic/thoracic; AI tissue alerting add-ons
Hugo RAS [3]	Medtronic	Vibrotactile + force feedback	Urology, gynaecology; AI-assisted instrument control
SPORT Surgical [4]	Titan Medical	6-DOF force feedback	Single-incision procedures; AI force prediction
Versius	CMR Surgical	Kinaesthetic resistance	General surgery; real-time AI performance analytics
Raven II (research)	Univ. Washington	Full force feedback	Open-source platform; RL-based haptic control
MAESTRO (research)	BioRobotics Lab	Multi-modal tactile	Microsurgery; AI tissue classification
Symani Surgical	MMI	Tremor filtering + force	Microsurgery <3 mm; AI-scale motion mapping

Overall, these platforms demonstrate the progression from basic haptic feedback to sophisticated AI-driven systems. Each platform leverages unique haptic modalities and AI capabilities to improve surgical safety, precision, and performance across various medical specialties.

4.1.1   AI-Driven Force-Feedback Restoration

AI-haptic systems restore the tactile channel in robotic surgery through two complementary strategies: direct measurement and predictive rendering [1]. Direct measurement embeds miniaturized force/torque sensors in the robotic instrument tip, transmitting measured contact forces back to the surgeon's hand controllers. The challenge is that instrument shaft resonances and friction in the port cannula corrupt the force signal; AI-based Kalman filters and 1-D CNN denoisers trained on intraoperative force profiles reconstruct the clean tissue contact force from the corrupted measurement. Predictive rendering addresses the problem that even after denoising, the electrical and mechanical transmission path introduces perceptible delay. Long short-term memory (LSTM) networks trained on annotated surgical procedure recordings predict tissue reaction forces 20–50 ms into the future [5], allowing the haptic controller to render predicted forces immediately and masking the true transmission latency below the threshold of perception. In laparoscopic cholecystectomy models, AI-haptic force restoration reduced inadvertent clipping force by 32% compared to standard robotic operation without haptic feedback.

4.1.2   Tissue Classification and Surgical Safety

Beyond force restoration, AI tissue classification provides a qualitatively new safety layer unavailable in conventional surgery. Convolutional neural networks trained on multispectral imaging and simultaneous force data classify tissue as parenchyma, vessel, nerve, or tumour margin in real time triggering differential haptic alert profiles that communicate the tissue identity through the surgeon's hand controllers without interrupting the surgical workflow [6]. In ex vivo porcine liver models, AI tissue classification achieved 94.7% accuracy at 30 Hz, sufficient for intraoperative deployment. Virtual fixtures, AI-enforced geometric no-go zones around critical structures identified in pre-operative CT/MRI prevent tool entry into danger regions through hard force barriers, supplemented by vibrotactile boundary alerts as the tool approaches the fixture boundary [1].

4.2   Medical Training and Simulation Systems

Medical simulation with haptic feedback addresses a fundamental challenge in surgical education: the ethical and logistical impossibility of practicing on patients until competence is demonstrated. Traditional apprenticeship models 'see one, do one, teach one's exposing patients to avoidable risk from novice trainees. High-fidelity haptic simulation offers a safe, reproducible environment for unlimited deliberate practice with objective performance measurement [7].

4.2.1   Patient-Specific Simulation

The highest-fidelity surgical simulators generate patient-specific virtual tissue models from pre-operative imaging data. U-Net segmentation applied to CT or MRI scans identifies organ boundaries, tumour locations, and vascular anatomy; this segmentation mesh is imported into a physics simulation engine (NVIDIA PhysX, SOFA Framework) that computes realistic tissue deformation, cutting, and suturing dynamics. AI models trained on ex vivo tissue mechanical testing data assign patient-appropriate elastic moduli, viscosities, and fracture thresholds to each tissue class, ensuring that the haptic simulation reflects the actual mechanical environment the surgeon will encounter [8].

Performance assessment AI analyses trainee interactions with the simulator across multiple dimensions: force application profiles (distinguishing confident, smooth manipulation from hesitant, jerky movements indicative of uncertainty), instrument trajectory efficiency (minimizing path length and tissue displacement), and error rate (inadvertent tissue contact, excessive force events). Explainable AI dashboards present these metrics visually, generating personalized feedback reports that identify specific technical deficits and recommend targeted practice scenarios [7].

Figure 4.2 illustrates the workflow of an AI-haptic medical simulation system. The process begins with pre-operative imaging, such as MRI or CT scans, which are used to

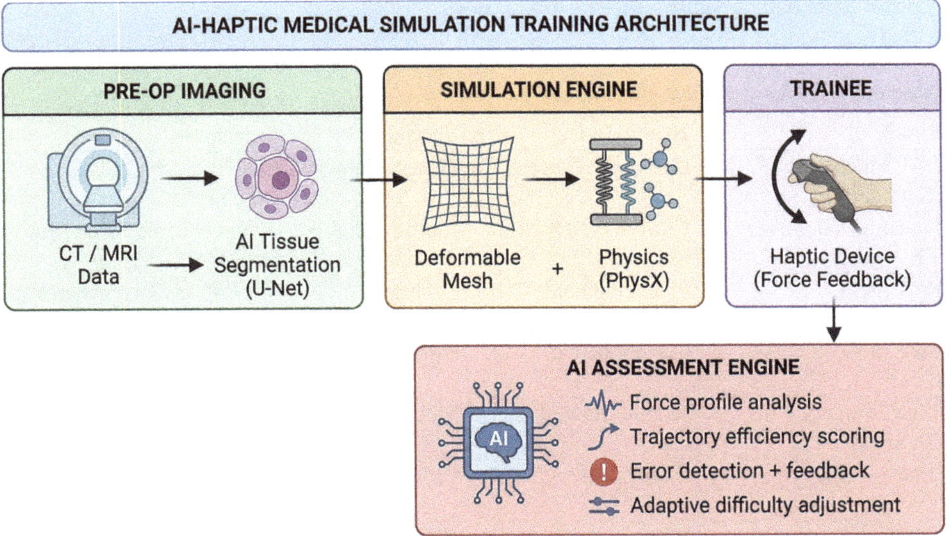

Fig. 4.2 Architecture of AI-haptic medical simulation system

create a digital model of the patient's anatomy. Next, AI algorithms perform tissue segmentation, identifying and separating different anatomical structures from the images. These segmented tissues are then used to generate a physics-based deformable mesh, which accurately simulates how tissues behave and respond to surgical manipulation. This mesh is integrated with haptic devices, allowing trainees to physically interact with the simulated tissues and experience realistic feedback. The system also includes an AI assessment engine, which evaluates trainee performance using several criteria: force profile analysis, trajectory efficiency scoring, error detection with feedback, and adaptive difficulty adjustment. This comprehensive architecture enables real-time, personalized training, helping trainees improve their skills through targeted feedback and scenario adaptation based on their competence level.

Table 4.2 summarizes various AI-powered haptic medical simulators, highlighting their areas of application (specialties), the type of haptic device they use, and the unique AI features integrated within each platform. These simulators are used in medical training to provide realistic, hands-on experience for trainees, helping them practice procedures safely and efficiently before working on real patients.

Below is a brief explanation of each simulator from the table:

- **LAP Mentor (Simbionix):** Used for general surgery training. It employs the Geomagic Touch+ haptic device to simulate real surgical tool handling and integrates AI for skill assessment and automatically adjusts the difficulty level as the user improves.
- **Fundamental Surgery VR:** A multi-speciality simulator uses a custom 6-degree-of-freedom arm. Its AI generates tissue models specific to each patient by analysing pre-operative CT scans, making practice more realistic and personalized.
- **ProstAsim:** Focused on urology, particularly prostate procedures. The Phantom Omni device simulates physical interactions, while AI creates accurate prostate tissue models from MRI data, enabling lifelike simulation.

Table 4.2 AI-haptic medical simulation platforms

Simulator	Haptic device	Speciality	AI features
LAP Mentor (Simbionix)	Geomagic Touch+	General surgery	AI skill scoring, adaptive difficulty
Fundamental Surgery VR	Custom 6-DOF arm	Multi-speciality	Patient-specific tissue from pre-op CT
ProstAsim	Phantom Omni	Urology	AI prostate tissue generation from MRI
EpiSim	Custom haptic	Anaesthesiology	Force feedback for epidural needle placement
Touch Surgery (DeSilva)	Mobile (limited haptic)	Multi-speciality	AI step detection, cognitive scoring
BoneTag VR	Haptic drill	Orthopaedics	AI bone density rendering from CT scan
CareSim	Vibrotactile glove	Nursing skills	AI assessment rubric, trainee analytics

- **EpiSim:** An anaesthesiology simulator that uses a custom haptic device to help trainees feel resistance and force when placing epidural needles. AI provides real-time force feedback for safe and precise needle placement.
- **Touch Surgery (DeSilva):** Covers multiple specialties with a mobile-based interface and limited haptic feedback. The AI tracks each step of the procedure, evaluates cognitive skills, and scores trainee performance.
- **BoneTag VR:** Designed for orthopaedics, especially bone-related procedures. The haptic drill simulates bone drilling, and AI processes CT scans to render bone density, making the tactile feedback match real patient anatomy.
- **CareSim:** Helps trainees develop nursing skills using a vibrotactile glove. AI analyses trainee actions against a detailed assessment rubric and offers analytics, identifying strengths and areas for improvement.

In summary, these platforms combine advanced haptic technology and artificial intelligence to deliver realistic, data-driven simulation experiences across a range of medical fields. The AI elements allow for personalization, objective skill measurement, and adaptive learning, ultimately improving trainee competence and patient safety.

4.2.2   Adaptive Difficulty and Curriculum Optimization

A key differentiator of AI-powered simulators over static scenario libraries is adaptive curriculum management. Bayesian knowledge tracing models maintain a probabilistic estimate of each trainee's current competence level across the surgical skill taxonomy, dynamically selecting the next simulation scenario that maximizes learning gain [9]. When a trainee consistently executes a task correctly, the AI increases difficulty by introducing anatomical variants, time pressure, or intraoperative complications (bleeding, adhesions). When performance degrades, difficulty is reduced and targeted remediation scenarios are presented. This closed-loop curriculum optimization has been shown to reduce the number of simulation hours required to achieve competency by 28–40% compared to fixed-sequence curricula.

4.3   Rehabilitation and Physical Therapy Applications

Neurological and musculoskeletal rehabilitation represents one of the largest and fastest growing markets for AI-haptic technology, driven by the global burden of stroke (15 million new cases annually), spinal cord injury, and traumatic orthopaedic conditions. AI-haptic rehabilitation systems address two complementary clinical goals, facilitating motor recovery through intensive, task-specific movement practice and providing real-time biofeedback that promotes neuroplasticity and correct movement pattern acquisition [10].

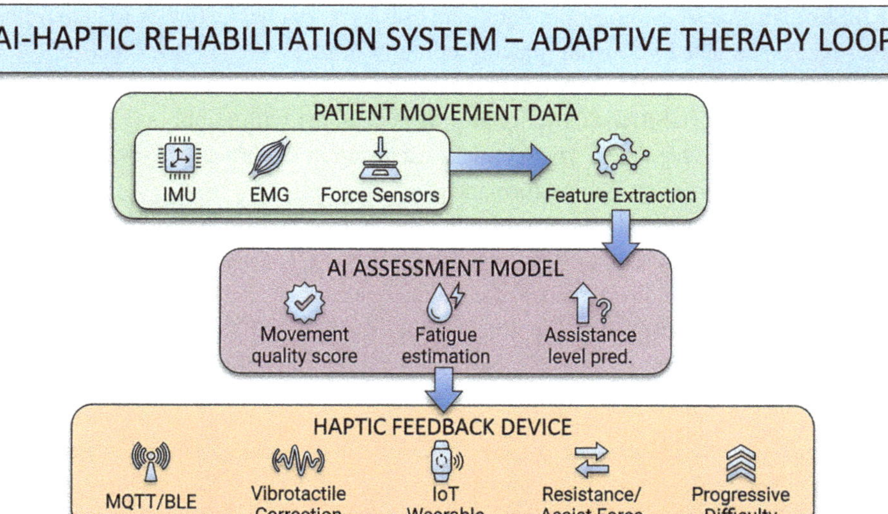

Fig. 4.3 AI-haptic rehabilitation adaptive therapy loop

Figure 4.3 illustrates the process by which a smart rehabilitation system uses artificial intelligence (AI) and haptic feedback to personalize therapy for patients. The loop begins with an Internet of Things (IoT) wearable device such as a sensor-equipped band or glove that collects real-time movement and muscle data from the patient during exercises. These sensor readings (for example, from IMU, EMG, or force sensors) are transmitted using MQTT (a lightweight messaging protocol suitable for IoT) to a cloud-based AI platform.

The AI system analyses the incoming sensor data to assess the patient's movement quality and determines the level of assistance or correction needed. Based on this assessment, the AI generates personalized commands for the haptic feedback device (such as a wearable with vibrotactile motors or resistance actuators). These commands are sent back to the wearable device, which delivers corrective cues like vibrations or resistance to guide the patient's movements, ensuring proper technique and progressive difficulty. This closed-loop system adapts therapy in real time, enhancing rehabilitation outcomes by providing timely and targeted feedback, and enabling therapy sessions to be conducted outside traditional clinical settings, such as in the patient's home.

Table 4.3 provides a comparative overview of advanced rehabilitation devices and platforms, focusing on four key aspects: the device or platform name, the specific medical condition treated, the type of haptic (touch-related) feedback modality used, and the AI capability integrated into each system. The table highlights how modern rehabilitation technologies combine haptic feedback and AI to personalize therapy, optimize movement, and enhance recovery for various neurological and musculoskeletal conditions. Devices use a range of touch-based or movement-based feedback, and AI capabilities help tailor interventions to each patient's needs, often adapting in real time as the patient progresses.

Table 4.3 AI-haptic rehabilitation systems

Device/Platform	Condition treated	Haptic modality	AI capability
Hocoma Armeo Power	Stroke, upper limb	Kinaesthetic exoskeleton	Adaptive assistance-as-needed control
ReWalk Exoskeleton	Spinal cord injury	Force-feedback gait assist	RL gait pattern optimisation
Hand of Hope (Rehab.)	Stroke hand function	EMG-triggered kinaesthetic	Intent detection, progressive difficulty
ReTouch Glove	Somatosensory deficits	Vibrotactile skin stimulation	AI sensory mapping personalisation
BioMex (DIH)	Post-stroke tremor	Impedance-controlled orthosis	Tremor classification and cancellation
CARES VR (Osso)	Post-surgical shoulder	Controller vibrotactile	AI exercise recognition + form scoring
InMotion ARM	Upper limb stroke	Planar kinaesthetic robot	Impedance adaptation via RL

4.3.1 Adaptive Assistance-as-Needed Control

The dominant AI control paradigm in robotic rehabilitation is assistance-as-needed (AAN): the robot provides just enough force assistance to complete the therapeutic movement, withdraw assistance as the patient's voluntary motor output increases [10]. Reinforcement learning agents trained on patient movement data learn to modulate assistance level continuously in response to intra-session fatigue, movement quality degradation, and task completion rate achieving the 'challenge point' of optimal motor learning more precisely than therapist-set manual resistance levels. In a randomized controlled trial of the InMotion ARM system, RL-based AAN control produced significantly greater Fugl-Meyer upper extremity improvements at 12 weeks compared to fixed-assistance robotic training. Vibrotactile biofeedback supplements motor assistance by conveying real-time movement quality information to patients with proprioceptive deficits, a common consequence of stroke affecting the parietal somatosensory cortex. Wearable vibrotactile arrays on the forearm encode joint angle deviations from the target trajectory as vibration patterns, providing an error signal that drives motor learning even in the absence of intact proprioception [9].

4.3.2 IoMT Integration for Remote Rehabilitation

The Internet of Medical Things (IoMT) enables rehabilitation AI-haptic systems to extend beyond clinical settings into the patient's home environment. MQTT-based communication protocols transmit sensor data (IMU, EMG, force) from wearable rehabilitation devices to cloud AI servers, which compute movement quality scores and adaptive exercise prescriptions [11]. Haptic feedback commands are transmitted back to the wearable device with sufficiently low latency (5–30 ms for non-time-critical movements) to provide corrective guidance during rehabilitation exercises. This architecture enables daily therapy sessions at home replacing the clinically established standard of twice-weekly outpatient physiotherapy and has demonstrated equivalent or superior motor outcomes in post-stroke upper limb rehabilitation trials when combined with AI-driven personalisation.

4.4   Smart Prosthetics and Assistive Technologies

Upper limb amputation affects over 1.5 million people globally, with myoelectric prostheses providing motor function restoration but historically offering no sensory feedback. The absence of tactile sensation forces prosthetic users to rely entirely on visual monitoring of the prosthetic hand, a cognitively demanding strategy that increases mental fatigue, reduces task performance, and contributes to prosthetic abandonment rates of 23–45% [12]. AI-haptic sensory restoration systems address this gap by creating a closed-loop tactile feedback channel from prosthetic fingertip sensors to the residual limb's peripheral nerves or the somatosensory cortex.

Figure 4.4 illustrates the process by which advanced prosthetic devices can recreate the sensation of touch for amputees. The system begins with a tactile sensor array embedded

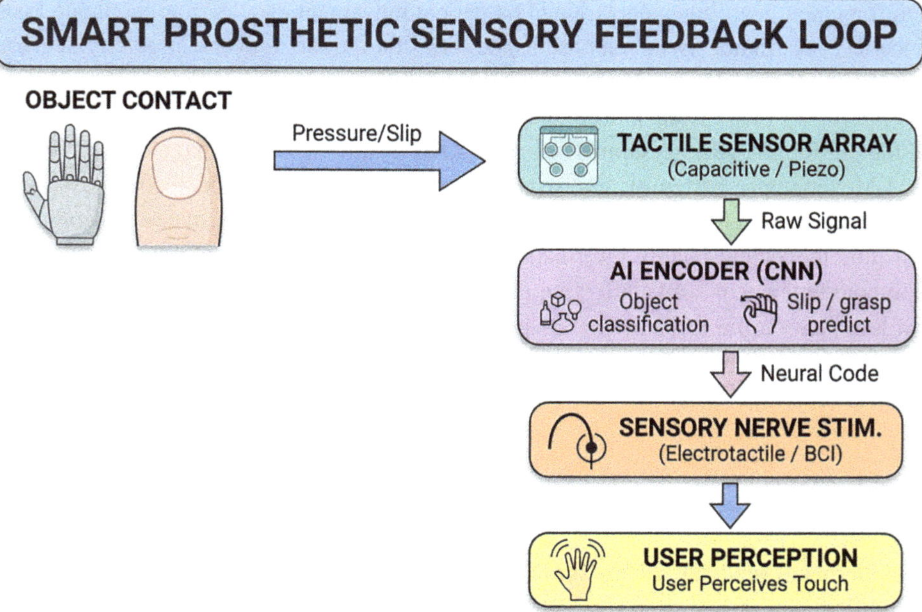

Fig. 4.4 Smart prosthetic sensory feedback loop

in the prosthetic limb, which detects physical contact, pressure, and other touch-related information. These raw sensory signals are then processed and classified by an AI encoder, which interprets the data and predicts important events such as slipping or securely grasping an object. The AI-processed signals are subsequently converted into neural codes that are used to stimulate the user's sensory nerves, either through electrotactile stimulation or brain–computer interface (BCI) technology. This sensory nerve stimulation allows the user to perceive tactile sensations as if they were feeling through a natural limb. The feedback loop enables the user to experience real-time touch, improving control, dexterity, and overall interaction with the environment.

Table 4.4 provides a comparative overview of leading smart prosthetic devices that leverage artificial intelligence (AI) to deliver advanced sensory feedback. Each row describes a specific device, its developer, the type of sensory feedback it provides, and the AI technologies integrated for enhanced user experience and function.

- **LUKE Arm (DEKA):** Developed by DEKA Research, this prosthetic provides both vibrotactile (touch-based) and proprioceptive (position sense) feedback. It uses AI-based pattern recognition of myoelectric signals (muscle activity) to enable intuitive control, allowing users to operate the arm more naturally.
- **i-Limb Ultra:** Manufactured by Össur, this device offers vibrotactile feedback. It employs AI algorithms to interpret electromyography (EMG) signals from the user's muscles, enabling the system to automatically select appropriate grip patterns for different tasks.
- **Psyonic Ability Hand:** Created by Psyonic, this hand features cutaneous vibrotactile feedback (skin-level touch sensations). Its AI integration consists of machine learning (ML) algorithms that adapt grip strength and patterns in real time based on touch sensor data, improving object handling.

Table 4.4 AI-enabled smart prosthetic devices

Device	Developer	Sensory feedback type	AI integration
LUKE Arm (DEKA) [13]	DEKA Research	Vibrotactile + proprioceptive	Pattern recognition myoelectric control
i-Limb Ultra [14]	Össur	Vibrotactile	AI grip selection from EMG patterns
Psyonic Ability Hand [15]	Psyonic	Cutaneous vibrotactile	Touch sensors + ML grip adaptation
BionIT Labs e-OPRA [16]	BionIT Labs	Osseoperception neural feedback	CNN decoding of tactile nerve signals
Modular Prosthetic Limb [17]	JHUAPL	Electrotactile stimulation	BCI with neural decoder for touch/slip
SmartHand (research) [18]	BioRobotics Inst.	Peripheral nerve stimulation.	AI tactile encoding for object identity
Orion BCI (Second Sight) [19]	Second Sight	Cortical visual stimulation	Deep learning retinal image encoding

- **BionIT Labs e-OPRA:** Developed by BionIT Labs, this prosthetic delivers osseoperception neural feedback, meaning it stimulates nerves via the bone-anchored implant to provide a sense of touch. Convolutional neural networks (CNNs) decode tactile nerve signals, translating sensor data into meaningful sensations for the user.
- **Modular Prosthetic Limb:** Built by the Johns Hopkins University Applied Physics Lab (JHUAPL), this limb uses electrotactile stimulation to mimic touch. It incorporates a brain–computer interface (BCI) with a neural decoder that enables users to perceive touch and slip events, enhancing control and responsiveness.
- **SmartHand (research):** Designed by the BioRobotics Institute, this research prototype uses peripheral nerve stimulation for sensory feedback. AI tactile encoding algorithms help identify object characteristics (such as texture or shape) via touch, providing more naturalistic sensation.
- **Orion BCI (Second Sight):** Developed by Second Sight, this device is unique as it focuses on vision restoration using cortical visual stimulation. Deep learning algorithms encode retinal images, which are then delivered to the brain via a brain–computer interface (BCI), allowing visually impaired users to perceive visual information.

4.4.1   Tactile Encoding and Neural Interfaces

The engineering challenge of somatosensory restoration is to translate the digital output of an artificial tactile sensor array into a neural stimulation pattern that the somatosensory cortex interprets as natural touch. Convolutional neural networks trained on neurophysiology datasets learn the mapping from physical contact parameters (normal force, shear, contact area, vibration frequency) to peripheral nerve firing rate patterns, generating stimulation pulse trains for electrotactile or peripheral nerve electrodes that mimic the afferent coding of natural mechanoreceptors [20].

In transcutaneous electrotactile systems used in the Psyonic Ability Hand and BionIT Labs e-OPRA platform, charge-controlled electrical pulses delivered to electrodes on the residual limb surface produce tactile sensations localized to the phantom hand through the cortical body map. AI models personalize the stimulation-to-sensation mapping for everyone, accounting for electrode placement variability, residual limb geometry, and perceptual threshold drift over time. Clinical studies report that electrotactile feedback reduces object drop rate by 47% and improves grooming and dressing task completion time by 31% [12].

4.4.2   Assistive Technologies for Visually Impaired Patients

Haptic technology extends beyond motor restoration to environmental navigation for visually impaired patients. Wearable haptic devices vibrotactile belts, wristbands, and vests translate spatial information from ultrasonic rangefinders, depth cameras, or computer vision systems into directional vibration patterns that guide users through complex environments [21]. AI semantic segmentation models identify obstacles, doorways, staircases, and wayfinding landmarks in depth images, encoding this spatial map as a vibrotactile body coordinate system that users learn to interpret through training. Hospital navigation systems using this architecture have demonstrated a 62% reduction in wayfinding errors for visually impaired patients navigating unfamiliar clinical environments, compared to standard cane techniques.

4.5   Telemedicine and Remote Healthcare Services

The COVID-19 pandemic accelerated telehealth adoption globally, exposing the fundamental limitation of video-only telemedicine: the absence of physical examination. Palpation, percussion, auscultation with simultaneous tissue palpation, and the tactile assessment of lymphadenopathy, organomegaly, and abdominal guarding are irreplaceable diagnostic acts that remote video consultation cannot approximate [22]. AI-haptic telemedicine systems are emerging as the technological response to this clinical gap, enabling remote physical examination through force-feedback haptic gloves connected to patient-side robotic palpation devices.

Figure 4.5 illustrates the architecture of a telemedicine haptic system designed for remote palpation, which enables clinicians to physically examine patients from a distance.

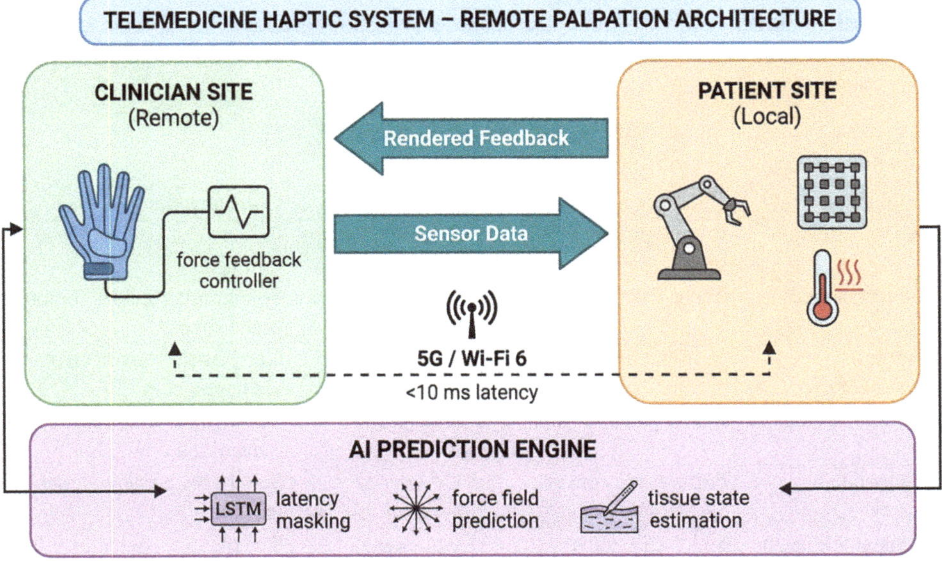

Fig. 4.5 Telemedicine haptic system for remote palpation

The system comprises four main components:

- **Clinician-site haptic controller:** This device allows healthcare professionals to perform palpation gestures, such as pressing or feeling, which are captured in real time.
- **Patient-site robotic palpation arm:** Located with the patient, this robotic arm replicates the clinician's movements, enabling remote physical interaction. The arm can apply force and sense tissue responses, providing feedback to the clinician.
- **5G communication layer:** High-speed 5G or Wi-Fi 6 networks transmit the control signals and sensor data between the clinician and patient sites. The low latency (less than 10 ms) is crucial for real-time, accurate haptic feedback, ensuring the clinician's actions are mirrored almost instantaneously.
- **AI prediction engine:** This module compensates for any communication delays by predicting the patient-site response using advanced algorithms such as LSTM (Long Short-Term Memory) latency masking. It also estimates force fields and tissue states, ensuring that the clinician receives timely and realistic feedback even if there are minor network interruptions.

Table 4.5 provides a comprehensive overview of various AI-driven haptic telemedicine applications, listing the specific devices used, the role of artificial intelligence in each, and their clinical benefits.

- **Remote palpation:** Uses a haptic glove paired with force/torque (F/T) sensors. AI algorithms provide predictive force rendering, which compensates for communication delays and enhances tactile feedback. Clinicians can remotely detect abnormalities like masses or tenderness in patients, closely simulating direct physical examination.
- **Tele-ultrasound:** A force-feedback probe allows sonographers to operate an ultrasound robot remotely. AI offers guidance by analysing images, ensuring accurate probe

Table 4.5 AI-haptic telemedicine applications

Application	Haptic device	AI role	Clinical value
Remote palpation	Haptic glove + F/T sensor	Predictive force rendering	Detects mass, tenderness remotely
Tele-ultrasound	Force-feedback probe	AI image guidance	Sonographer guides remote probe robot
Remote physiotherapy	Vibrotactile wristband	RL exercise adaptation	Corrects movement errors via haptic cues
Tele-dermatology	e-Skin patch	AI texture classification	Lesion hardness/texture transmitted remotely
Teleoperated surgery	Full robotic console	LSTM latency compensation	Sub-10 ms perceptual delay masking
Neonatal tele-exam	Soft tactile glove	AI vital-sign estimation	Remote assessment of fontanelle tension
Remote dental exam	Haptic dental probe	AI caries detection	Tactile mapping of tooth surface remotely

placement. This enables remote scanning, with a level of diagnostic precision comparable to in-person ultrasound.

- **Remote physiotherapy:** Vibrotactile wristbands provide haptic cues to patients during exercises. Reinforcement learning (RL) algorithms adapt the exercise regimen based on movement feedback, correcting errors and improving rehabilitation outcomes even when sessions are conducted remotely.
- **Tele-dermatology:** Electronic skin (e-skin) patches collect data about skin texture and hardness. AI classifies these tactile properties, allowing dermatologists to remotely assess lesions, rashes, or other skin conditions with a tactile sense like in-person assessment.
- **Teleoperated surgery:** Surgeons use a full robotic console with haptic feedback. AI, specifically Long Short-Term Memory (LSTM) models, compensate for latency, ensuring that the surgeon's actions and feedback are nearly instantaneous. This technology masks perceptual delays to below 10 ms, which is crucial for delicate surgical procedures performed remotely.
- **Neonatal tele-exam:** Soft tactile gloves are used to remotely assess newborns. AI estimates vital signs by interpreting tactile data, enabling clinicians to evaluate conditions like fontanelle tension (soft spot on the infant's head) without direct contact, which is especially valuable for neonatal care in distant locations.
- **Remote dental exam:** Haptic dental probes are manipulated by clinicians to examine tooth surfaces remotely. AI detects dental caries (cavities) and provides tactile mapping, allowing dentists to perform thorough dental assessments even when the patient is not physically present.

Overall, the table highlights how AI and haptic technologies are transforming telemedicine by providing remote clinicians with tactile feedback and diagnostic capabilities that were previously only possible through direct physical contact. This advancement bridges the gap in remote healthcare, enabling high-quality examinations, treatments, and procedures from a distance and improving access and outcomes across various medical fields.

4.5.1 Remote Palpation and Tele-Examination

A remote palpation system comprises three core components: a patient-side robotic palpation device equipped with force/torque sensors and a compliance-controlled end-effector; a clinician-side haptic interface (force-feedback glove or robotic arm controller); and an AI latency compensation layer that masks communication delay [22]. The clinician applies palpation pressure through the haptic controller; the command is transmitted to the patient-side robot, which applies the corresponding force to the patient's abdomen, chest, or lymph node region. Sensor readings are transmitted back and rendered on the clinician's haptic device, recreating the tactile sensation of direct palpation. Over 5G networks with round-trip latencies of 10–20 ms, LSTM predictive haptic rendering effectively masks the delay, achieving a haptic realism score of 7.2/10 in clinician evaluation studies compared to 8.4/10 for direct palpation and 3.1/10 for remote palpation without AI latency compensation [5]. Tele-ultrasound, combining AI-guided probe positioning with force feedback on the sonographer's remote controller, has demonstrated diagnostic accuracy for obstetric, cardiac, and abdominal imaging comparable to in-person examination in controlled clinical trials.

4.5.2 Haptic Alerts for Healthcare Workers

A distinct telemedicine application involves haptic alerting for healthcare workers operating in environments where visual and auditory attention are occupied. Clinical nurses, theatre practitioners, and emergency response staff wear haptic wristbands or pager-integrated vibrotactile devices that encode alert priority through vibration intensity and pattern: a single short pulse for routine notifications, escalating frequency patterns for urgent alerts, and continuous strong vibration for critical emergency calls. AI context awareness models trained on hospital workflow patterns and integrated with electronic patient monitoring systems determine alert priority levels and modality routing in real time, reducing alarm fatigue by filtering non-actionable alerts before haptic delivery.

4.6   Pain Management and Sensory Therapy

Pain management represents an underexplored but clinically significant application domain for AI-haptic technology. The gate control theory of pain which proposes that non-nociceptive tactile stimulation can inhibit pain signal transmission at the dorsal horn of the spinal cord provides the biophysical rationale for vibrotactile and TENS-based haptic analgesia. AI systems that optimize stimulation parameters in real time based on patient-reported pain scores and physiological signals (heart rate variability, skin conductance, facial expression) extend this principle into adaptive, personalized pain management.

4.6.1 VR-Haptic Pain Distraction

Virtual reality combined with haptic feedback has demonstrated significant analgesic efficacy in acute pain scenarios particularly burns dressing changes, which involve repeated high-intensity procedural pain that poorly responds to pharmacological analgesia alone [23]. Immersive VR environments (Snow World, developed at the University of Washington) reduce procedural pain scores by an average of 3.5 points on the NRS scale comparable to opioid analgesic effect sizes by competing with nociceptive signals for attentional resources. AI systems that monitor physiological stress indicators and dynamically adjust VR immersion depth and haptic sensory engagement level maintain optimal analgesic effect throughout the procedure.

4.6.2   Phantom Limb Pain Management

Phantom limb pain experienced by 60–80% of amputees arise from maladaptive cortical reorganization following limb loss. Mirror therapy, which uses visual illusion of the intact limb to normalize cortical body maps, is the established first-line intervention; AI-haptic systems extend this approach by providing vibrotactile stimulation to the residual limb synchronized with virtual limb movements in an augmented reality environment [12]. Reinforcement learning agents personalize the stimulation pattern and AR illusion parameters for each patient, optimizing for pain reduction outcomes reported at each session.

4.7   Case Studies in AI-Haptic Healthcare

This section presents detailed real-world use cases drawn from clinical practice and applied research, illustrating the practical implementation of AI-haptic systems across the key application domains examined in this chapter. The use cases are structured according to the Haptic Communication in Healthcare framework, which identifies five primary communication objectives: remote consultation, rehabilitation support, alerts for healthcare providers, guidance for surgical procedures, and assistive technology for visually impaired patients.

4.7.1   Remote Consultation with Haptic Devices

- **Application:** Haptic-enabled systems allow clinicians to remotely assess patients by simulating the tactile experience of palpation, pulse assessment, and interactive navigation through three-dimensional virtual patient models. This creates a more immersive telemedicine environment, bridging the sensory gap between remote and in-person care.
- **Implementation:** Development of advanced haptic gloves or peripheral devices that transmit real-time tactile feedback to healthcare providers, enhancing the fidelity and diagnostic value of remote examinations.

4.7.2   Rehabilitation Supported by Haptic Feedback

- **Application:** Patients undergoing rehabilitation benefit from wearable haptic devices that provide real-time feedback during therapeutic exercises. These cues help ensure correct movement patterns and enhance engagement in home-based or supervised rehabilitation programmes.
- **Implementation:** Integration of vibrotactile or pressure-based wearables that guide and correct patient movements, fostering more effective and adaptive rehabilitation outcomes.

4.7.3 Haptic Alerts for Healthcare Workers

- **Application:** Haptic alerting systems deliver discrete, prioritized notifications to healthcare professionals such as nurses and emergency staff when visual and auditory channels are saturated. Vibration patterns and intensities are mapped to alert urgency, ensuring critical messages are received promptly without adding to alarm fatigue.
- **Implementation:** Deployment of wristbands or pager-integrated wearables that differentiate alert types through distinctive vibration signatures, managed by AI-driven workflow and patient monitoring systems that filter and prioritize alerts in real time.

4.7.4 Haptic Guidance for Surgical Procedures

- **Application:** Surgeons performing minimally invasive operations can receive real-time tactile cues about anatomical structures and instrument interactions, enhancing spatial awareness and precision during complex procedures.
- **Implementation:** Integration of haptic feedback modules within surgical tools, allowing for dynamic, context-sensitive tactile information to be delivered during live surgery.

4.7.5 Assistive Haptic Technologies for Visually Impaired Patients

- **Application:** Visually impaired individuals can navigate complex hospital environments more independently with the support of haptic guidance systems, which deliver navigational cues through wearable devices.
- **Implementation:** Use of wearable haptic interfaces such as belts or wristbands that communicate direction and proximity information via vibratory patterns, enhancing safe and efficient mobility within healthcare facilities.

4.8 Practical Examples in AI-Haptic Healthcare

This section presents practical example for AI-driven haptic guidance in surgical systems and rehabilitation with haptic feedback with codes.

4.8.1   A Predictive Framework for AI-Driven Haptic Guidance in Surgical Systems

The integration of the Internet of Medical Things (IoMT) and Artificial Intelligence (AI) is catalysing a digital transformation in surgical practices. By combining real-time data acquisition with predictive analytics and haptic feedback, a new class of 'smart' surgical systems is emerging. These systems do not merely automate tasks but provide a sophisticated guidance layer that enhances human precision and decision-making.

- **System Architecture and Implementation**

- To develop a predictive model for haptic guidance, the system must be built upon a multi-layered architecture:

  - **Data Acquisition and Integration:** The foundation involves utilizing sensors, actuators, and IoT devices to capture a vast array of data from both surgical environments and patients. This includes implementing smart wearables to monitor patient health data continuously.
  - **Haptic Feedback Technology:** The system employs haptic interfaces that provide tactile and force feedback to surgeons, improving spatial awareness and precision. This integration, including haptic gloves, enables surgeons to 'feel' internal environments without direct physical contact.
  - **Machine Learning and Predictive Analytics:** Algorithms analyse real-time and historical data to predict surgical outcomes. Predictive models anticipate potential challenges or changes in patient status, facilitating more informed decision-making.
  - **Network and Communication:** Secure, real-time communication networks are established to ensure immediate data transmission between IoT devices. Edge computing is implemented to process data closer to its source, significantly reducing latency.
  - **Real-time Decision Guidance:** The AI processes incoming data to offer insights through haptic, visual, and auditory signals. The model can guide manoeuvres and suggest alternative strategies when unexpected scenarios occur.
  - **Security, Compliance, and Adaptation:** Robust cybersecurity protocols protect sensitive patient data within the IoMT network while adhering to healthcare regulations. Furthermore, adaptive learning algorithms allow the system to continuously improve from every procedure.

- **Potential Clinical Applications**
- This framework enables several transformative applications in modern medicine:

  - **Remote Surgeries:** Haptic feedback allows surgeons to conduct procedures from a distance, experiencing tactile sensations as if physically present at the bedside.

- **Training and Simulation:** Medical professionals can utilize realistic haptic environments to practice complex procedures in a risk-free virtual space.
- **Enhanced Precision and Safety:** By predicting complications and providing alternative strategies, the model minimizes procedural risks and enhances precision.
- **Postoperative and Personalized Care:** IoMT devices provide continuous monitoring post-surgery to prevent complications, while the accumulated data helps create personalized recovery trajectories for each patient.

- **Challenges and Future Considerations**

- Despite its potential, several hurdles remain for widespread adoption:

  - **Privacy and Security:** Protecting patient data in a highly connected IoMT environment is a critical priority.
  - **System Integration:** New technologies must be designed to integrate seamlessly with existing healthcare infrastructures and clinical protocols.
  - **Reliability and Trust:** For healthcare professionals to adopt these tools, the systems must demonstrate near-perfect accuracy and reliability.
  - **Regulatory and Economic Barriers:** Navigating the complex landscape of regulatory approval and ensuring that the technology is cost-effective are essential for accessibility.

- **Technical Workflow: Model Training and Communication Protocols**

- The operational efficiency of a predictive haptic guidance system relies on a seamless loop between the edge device (surgical tool), the communication protocol, and the centralized AI server.

  - **Training of the Model:** Using an AI classifier, the system can make autonomous or semi-autonomous decisions about proceeding with a surgery based on synthetic data. This allows the model to be pre-trained on diverse surgical scenarios including rare complications before encountering real-world patient data.

```python
import pandas as pd
import numpy as np
import random
from sklearn.tree import DecisionTreeClassifier
from sklearn.model_selection import train_test_split
from sklearn.metrics import accuracy_score
import joblib

# Generate synthetic data (as in the previous example)
num_samples = 10000
data = {
    'force': np.random.uniform(0, 100, num_samples),
    'vibration': np.random.uniform(0, 1, num_samples),
    'torque': np.random.uniform(0, 100, num_samples),
    'position_x': np.random.uniform(-100, 100, num_samples),
    'position_y': np.random.uniform(-100, 100, num_samples),
    'position_z': np.random.uniform(-100, 100, num_samples),
    'velocity': np.random.uniform(0, 100, num_samples),
    'acceleration': np.random.uniform(0, 100, num_samples),
    'decision': [random.choice(['Proceed', 'Proceed with caution', 'Delay', 'Second Opinion',
'Not Confident'])
                 for _ in range(num_samples)]
}
df = pd.DataFrame(data)

# Prepare data for training
X = df.drop('decision', axis=1)
y = df['decision']
X_train, X_test, y_train, y_test = train_test_split(X, y, test_size=0.2, random_state=42)

# Train a Decision Tree model
model = DecisionTreeClassifier(random_state=55)
model.fit(X_train, y_train)

# Evaluate the model
predictions = model.predict(X_test)
accuracy = accuracy_score(y_test, predictions)
print(f'Model Accuracy: {accuracy*100:.0f}%')

# Save the model
joblib.dump(model, 'surgery_decision_model.pkl')

# Load the model and make a prediction
loaded_model = joblib.load('surgery_decision_model.pkl')
sample_input = np.array([20, 0.5, 30, -50, 40, 60, 10, 15]).reshape(1, -1)
prediction = loaded_model.predict(sample_input)[0]
print(f'Model Prediction: {prediction}')
```

- **Device Side (Data Ingestion):** Using industry-standard protocols like **MQTT (Message Queuing Telemetry Transport)**, an IoT-enabled surgical device captures and transmits high-frequency telemetry. Key data streams include:

  Kinetic Data: Force, vibration, and torque applied to tissue.

  Kinematic Data: Spatial position coordinates (x, y, z), velocity, and acceleration of the instrument tip.

```python
# Device Side

import paho.mqtt.client as mqtt
import json
import numpy as np
import time


# Callback when a message is received
def on_message(client, userdata, msg):
    decision = msg.payload.decode('utf-8')
    print(f"Decision Received from Server: {decision}")

client = mqtt.Client()
client.on_message = on_message

# Connect to the broker
client.connect("broker.hivemq.com", 1883, 60)

# Subscribe to the topic to receive decisions
client.subscribe("IOMT/surgery/decision")

client.loop_start()

try:
    while True:
        # Generate a synthetic sample - replace with actual sensor readings in a real imple-
mentation
        sample_input = np.random.uniform(-100, 100, 8).tolist()
        client.publish("IOMT/surgery/input", json.dumps({'data': sample_input}))

        # Wait for a few seconds before sending the next sample
        time.sleep(5)
except KeyboardInterrupt:
    pass
finally:
    client.loop_stop()
    client.disconnect()
```

- **Server Side (Processing and Prediction):** The server acts as a listener, constantly monitoring incoming MQTT topics for new telemetry. Upon receipt, the pre-trained classifier processes the data to:

  Predict the current surgical state or potential hazards.
  Transmit prediction information back to the user interface or haptic actuator.

```python
import paho.mqtt.client as mqtt
import json
import joblib
import numpy as np

# Load the trained model
model = joblib.load('surgery_decision_model.pkl')

# Callback when a message is received
def on_message(client, userdata, msg):
    input_data = json.loads(msg.payload.decode('utf-8'))['data']
    prediction = model.predict(np.array(input_data).reshape(1, -1))[0]
    # Displaying received data and prediction on the server-side
    print(f"Received data: {input_data}")
    print(f"Prediction by Model: {prediction}")
    client.publish("IOMT/surgery/decision", prediction)

client = mqtt.Client()
client.on_message = on_message

# Connect to the broker
client.connect("broker.hivemq.com", 1883, 60)

# Subscribe to the topic to receive sensor readings
client.subscribe("IOMT/surgery/input")

client.loop_forever()
```

System Output and Logic

The following logic outlines the data flow between the hardware and software layers:

- **Device Output:** The IoT device generates a continuous stream of telemetry packets.

Received data: [-19.4428226050118, -4.065801694346121, -23.476872712242994, 15.075608574788973, 69.89867895669332, 12.092580495895959, -63.82526019587165, -99.47939224615277]

Prediction by Model: Second Opinion

Received data: [-24.160162633441345, -16.579003274055765, -0.9760206366718762, 82.74455469416034, 60.17516317560819, -31.966099083166483, 36.58217540252855, -39.564177125239006]

Prediction by Model: Second Opinion

Received data: [-91.10891708889473, -78.13767319996717, -11.252183837950724, -30.68025431324824, -17.830082381313517, -90.45861312453746, -30.86728184056919, 65.58951851149675]

Prediction by Model: Second Opinion

Received data: [-21.10861824301631, -32.835395272179, 2.260337801517508, 91.30471061915989, -40.88888949534033, 45.970354246890224, 4.995947355202944, 53.035444524056146]

Prediction by Model: Proceed with caution

Received data: [-31.57836199139578, -48.2635313915712, -66.40309183111646, -24.146748635437405, -99.80713962334156, -55.484792311148865, -80.31133025276587, 34.74655893840591]

Prediction by Model: Proceed

Received data: [-73.54135869254775, -24.305635178444845, -70.69339589835747, 85.11157841009907, 24.09070753378964, -86.88350069863948, -61.632690965442926, 61.55851273999977]

Prediction by Model: Proceed with caution

Received data: [-23.855651743857905, 47.90983420406721, 26.20197821686159, 63.96055652516816, 84.81075740501467, -89.98282597589251, -81.11680415442692, -20.745458417902654]

Prediction by Model: Proceed

Received data: [73.89042690543721, -75.52345348311076, 0.01481433744095284, 32.497321197165604, 14.103261784320978, 43.416942899434474, -28.9055321393662, -43.10931201187906]

Prediction by Model: Delay

Received data: [-45.12918765148761, -25.542700386854662, -21.2334107391235, 6.01729561097433, -50.023908667132446, 19.350893339558, -45.64591049138711, -44.16224605393626]

Prediction by Model: Second Opinion

- **Predictive Output:** The server-side model outputs a decision variable (e.g. 'Safe to Proceed', 'Resistance Detected', or 'Deviation Warning').

Decision Received from Server: Second Opinion

Decision Received from Server: Second Opinion

Decision Received from Server: Second Opinion

Decision Received from Server: Proceed with caution

Decision Received from Server: Proceed

Decision Received from Server: Proceed with caution

Decision Received from Server: Proceed

Decision Received from Server: Delay

Decision Received from Server: Second Opinion

- **User Feedback:** The prediction is translated into haptic resistance or visual alerts, closing the loop of the haptic guidance system.

4.8.2   A Predictive Framework for Neurorehabilitation and Haptic Feedback Systems

Predictive modelling in rehabilitation involves the strategic application of technology to anticipate and facilitate the recovery trajectories of individuals undergoing therapeutic interventions. This multidisciplinary approach blends physical therapy with technological innovations, specifically targeting the tactile sense to enhance the efficacy of skill acquisition and motor learning.

- **Theoretical Foundations of Haptic Interaction**

- Haptic feedback serves as a critical bridge between digital intelligence and physical recovery.

  - **Mechanism of Action:** These systems leverage the sense of touch by applying precisely calibrated forces, vibrations, or motions to the user via wearable or robotic interfaces.
  - **Therapeutic Importance:** In a rehabilitative context, haptics provides **real**-time tactile responses that guide the neuroplasticity process, ensuring the patient adheres to optimal movement patterns.

- **Enabling Technologies and Tools**
- The implementation of this framework relies on a specialized technological stack:

  - **Wearable Devices:** High-fidelity gloves and suits are utilized to provide sensory substitution or augmentation, assisting in motor learning.

- **Robotic Systems:** Exoskeletons and end-effector robots guide patient limbs through specific trajectories, providing supportive 'assistance-as-needed' force.
- **Immersive Virtual Reality (VR):** VR environments coupled with haptic controllers create engaging, gamified therapy sessions that increase patient motivation and adherence.

- **Intelligence and Personalization Through AI**
- Predictive modelling transforms rehabilitation from a reactive process to a proactive one by leveraging data-driven insights.

  - **Data Synthesis:** Systems collect high-resolution data regarding movement kinematics, strength, and physiological progress.
  - **Machine Learning and AI:** Advanced algorithms, including Reinforcement Learning (RL), analyse these datasets to discern patterns and predict optimal rehabilitation pathways.
  - **Dynamic Personalization:** Predictive models facilitate a tailor-made approach that evolves in real time as the patient recovers, adjusting the level of robot-assisted force based on current performance.

- **Technical Implementation and Communication Architecture**
- The practical execution of a predictive rehabilitation model follows a structured IoT-based workflow.

  - **AI Model Training**

  - The core intelligence is often a classifier trained to predict the required level of assistance.
    Predictive Logic: Using sensor data, the AI determines whether to increase or decrease robotic support (e.g. assistance-as-needed).
    Data Sources: Training often utilizes synthetic data and historical patient logs to ensure robust prediction across varying levels of impairment.

```python
import numpy as np
from sklearn.model_selection import train_test_split
from sklearn.ensemble import RandomForestRegressor
from sklearn.metrics import mean_squared_error
import joblib

# Seed for reproducibility
np.random.seed(0)

# Generate synthetic data
X = np.random.rand(100, 5)   # 100 samples, 5 features representing sensor readings

# Ensure y is in the range [0, 100] to represent percentage
# Note: This is a simplistic way to get percentages and might not be valid in real-world ap-
plications
y = np.random.rand(100) * 100

# Split the data
X_train, X_test, y_train, y_test = train_test_split(X, y, test_size=0.2, random_state=0)

# Train a model
model = RandomForestRegressor(random_state=0)
model.fit(X_train, y_train)

# Evaluate the model
predictions = model.predict(X_test)
mse = mean_squared_error(y_test, predictions)
print(f"Mean Squared Error: {mse}")

# Save the model
joblib.dump(model, 'haptic_model.joblib')

# Usage in a hypothetical rehabilitation scenario
new_data = np.array([0.5, 0.3, 0.7, 0.8, 0.2]).reshape(1, -1)
predicted_assistance = model.predict(new_data)[0]

# Provide feedback: Predicted percentage might inform the level of haptic feedback or assis-
tance needed.
print(f"Predicted Level of Assistance Needed: {predicted_assistance:.2f}%")
```

Output: Trained AI models used to predict the percentage of assistance needed.

Mean Squared Error: 1190.5894197453777

Predicted Level of Assistance Needed: 64.87%

- **Device-Side Data Ingestion (Edge Layer)**
- The physical rehabilitation device acts as an IoT edge node.
    Communication Protocols: Using lightweight protocols like MQTT, the device transmits real-time telemetry including force, position coordinates, and velocity to a central server.

```python
import paho.mqtt.client as mqtt
import numpy as np
import time
import json

# MQTT settings
BROKER = "broker.hivemq.com"
PORT = 1883
TOPIC = "haptic/sensor_data"

client = mqtt.Client("Device")

# Connect to the broker
client.connect(BROKER, PORT)

# Generate and send synthetic sensor data
while True:
    # Example: Generate random synthetic sensor data
    sensor_data = np.random.rand(1, 5).tolist()

    # Convert data to JSON and publish it
    client.publish(TOPIC, json.dumps({"sensor_data": sensor_data}), qos=1)

    # Display message
    print(f"Sent sensor data: {sensor_data}")

    # Wait before sending next data point
    time.sleep(1)
```

Output: A continuous stream of sensory packets representing the patient's physical state.

Sent sensor data: [[0.5765565010832875, 0.7727146355648674, 0.8700069705495137, 0.2551815827404291, 0.5678458199820866]]

Sent sensor data: [[0.3645806173911228, 0.9683692377936935, 0.0440619082713567, 0.013110285320632409, 0.14998909643559077]]

Sent sensor data: [[0.3738611005266729, 0.34583613328989626, 0.13799504780488903, 0.9902114353892192, 0.8374411037175464]]

Sent sensor data: [[0.22422004209318724, 0.05930332295168894, 0.6318440002811576, 0.46754923784312796, 0.482709891840587]]

Sent sensor data: [[0.5831308842240241, 0.24492348364873395, 0.10111674820936489, 0.28856969414678046, 0.04914668837494374]]

Sent sensor data: [[0.7652805063086704, 0.6130520462496601, 0.3594732729177913, 0.8366646884800908, 0.41899334921891485]]

- **Server-Side Prediction (Cloud/Local Server)**

- The server processes incoming data to close the therapeutic loop.

    Real-time Processing: The server listens for incoming MQTT messages and executes the trained model.

```python
import paho.mqtt.client as mqtt
import json
import joblib
import numpy as np

# Load the pre-trained model
# Ensure you have a trained model saved as 'haptic_model.joblib'
model = joblib.load('haptic_model.joblib')

# MQTT settings
BROKER = "broker.hivemq.com"
PORT = 1883
TOPIC = "haptic/sensor_data"


# Callback function to handle received messages
def on_message(client, userdata, message):
    # Decode message and extract sensor data
    msg = json.loads(message.payload.decode())
    sensor_data = np.array(msg["sensor_data"])

    # Predict the level of assistance needed using the model
    predicted_assistance = model.predict(sensor_data)[0]

    # Display received message and prediction
    print(f"Received sensor data: {sensor_data}")
    print(f"Predicted Level of Assistance Needed: {predicted_assistance:.2f}%")

# Set up MQTT client
client = mqtt.Client("Server")
client.connect(BROKER, PORT)

# Specify callback function and subscribe to topic
client.on_message = on_message
client.subscribe(TOPIC)

# Start listening
try:
    print("Server is listening for incoming messages...")
    client.loop_forever()
except KeyboardInterrupt:
    print("\nServer stopped.")
```

Decision Output: The model predicts the necessary intervention and transmits the command back to the device to adjust haptic feedback levels immediately.

Server is listening for incoming messages...

Received sensor data: [[0.5765565 0.77271464 0.87000697 0.25518158 0.56784582]]

Predicted Level of Assistance Needed: 54.98%

Received sensor data: [[0.36458062 0.96836924 0.04406191 0.01311029 0.1499891]]

Predicted Level of Assistance Needed: 37.45%

Received sensor data: [[0.3738611 0.34583613 0.13799505 0.99021144 0.8374411]]

Predicted Level of Assistance Needed: 46.28%

Received sensor data: [[0.22422004 0.05930332 0.631844   0.46754924 0.48270989]]

Predicted Level of Assistance Needed: 65.67%

Received sensor data: [[0.58313088 0.24492348 0.10111675 0.28856969 0.04914669]]

Predicted Level of Assistance Needed: 53.62%

- **Clinical Considerations and Future Directions**

- While the benefits include enhanced precision, increased engagement, and the potential for remote therapy, several challenges must be addressed:

  - **Accessibility and Safety:** Ensuring devices are ergonomic, comfortable, and usable for patients across different age groups and tech proficiencies.
  - **Data Ethics:** Maintaining strict confidentiality and security for sensitive patient movement data within the IoMT network.
  - **Clinical Validation:** Ongoing research in stroke and musculoskeletal rehabilitation continues to refine how haptic-guided systems optimize posture and strength recovery.

4.9 Summary

This chapter provides the clinical translation of AI-powered haptic technology, illustrating how tactile feedback integrated with machine learning addresses critical gaps in modern healthcare. In the realm of robotic minimally invasive surgery, AI systems combat the 'haptic deficit'—the lack of physical sensation for the surgeon—through strategies like direct sensor measurement and predictive rendering, which uses Long Short-Term Memory (LSTM) networks to mask communication latency. These platforms, including the da Vinci Xi and Hugo RAS, leverage convolutional neural networks for real-time tissue classification, allowing the system to identify parenchyma, vessels, or nerves and provide differential haptic alerts to improve surgical safety.

Beyond the operating room, AI-driven haptic simulation provides a high-fidelity training environment where trainees can practice complex procedures on patient-specific virtual models generated from pre-operative CT or MRI scans. These systems utilize physics engines like NVIDIA PhysX to simulate realistic tissue deformation and employ Bayesian knowledge tracing to dynamically adjust the curriculum based on a trainee's evolving competence. Similarly, in rehabilitation, AI-haptic platforms for stroke and musculoskeletal recovery utilize 'assistance-as-needed' (AAN) control. In this closed-loop architecture, reinforcement learning agents monitor patient movement and fatigue via IoT wearables, providing real-time vibrotactile biofeedback or robotic assistance to optimize neuroplasticity and motor learning.

Technology also offers transformative solutions for sensory restoration and remote care. Smart prosthetics, such as the LUKE Arm and i-Limb Ultra, use AI encoders to translate prosthetic sensor data into neural codes, restoring a sense of touch to amputees and reducing object drop rates. In telemedicine, the integration of 5G networks and AI prediction engines enables remote physical examinations, allowing clinicians to 'feel' a patient's tissue via haptic gloves and robotic arms with sub-10 ms perceived latency. Furthermore, AI-haptic modalities are being applied to pain management through VR-haptic distraction and to assist visually impaired patients in navigating complex hospital environments using directional vibration patterns. Despite these advancements, the chapter notes that widespread adoption faces challenges regarding data security within the Internet of Medical Things (IoMT), system reliability, and regulatory hurdles.

References

1. Okamura, A. M. (2009). Haptic feedback in robot-assisted minimally invasive surgery. *Current Opinion in Urology, 19*(1), 102–107.
2. DiMaio, S., Hanuschik, M., & Kreaden, U. (2010). The da Vinci surgical system. In *Surgical robotics: Systems applications and visions* (pp. 199–217). Springer US.
3. Totaro, A., Scarciglia, E., Marino, F., Campetella, M., Gandi, C., Ragonese, M., et al. (2024). Robot-assisted radical prostatectomy performed with the novel surgical robotic platform Hugo™ RAS: Monocentric first series of 132 cases reporting surgical, and early functional and oncological outcomes at a tertiary referral robotic center. *Cancers, 16*(8), 1602.
4. Seeliger, B., Diana, M., Ruurda, J. P., Konstantinidis, K. M., Marescaux, J., & Swanström, L. L. (2019). Enabling single-site laparoscopy: The SPORT platform. *Surgical Endoscopy, 33*(11), 3696–3703.
5. Hochreiter, S., & Schmidhuber, J. (1997). Long short-term memory. *Neural Computation, 9*(8), 1735–1780.
6. Topol, E. J. (2019). High-performance medicine: The convergence of human and artificial intelligence. *Nature Medicine, 25*(1), 44–56.
7. Riek, L. D. (2017). Healthcare robotics. *Communications of the ACM, 60*(11), 68–78.
8. Raissi, M., Perdikaris, P., & Karniadakis, G. E. (2019). Physics-informed neural networks: A deep learning framework for solving forward and inverse problems involving nonlinear partial differential equations. *Journal of Computational Physics, 378*, 686–707.
9. Finn, C., Abbeel, P., & Levine, S. (2017, July). Model-agnostic meta-learning for fast adaptation of deep networks. In *International conference on machine learning* (pp. 1126–1135). PMLR.
10. Marchal-Crespo, L., & Reinkensmeyer, D. J. (2009). Review of control strategies for robotic movement training after neurologic injury. *Journal of Neuroengineering and Rehabilitation, 6*(1), 20.
11. Shi, W., Cao, J., Zhang, Q., Li, Y., & Xu, L. (2016). Edge computing: Vision and challenges. *IEEE Internet of Things Journal, 3*(5), 637–646.
12. Lotze, M., Grodd, W., Birbaumer, N., Erb, M., Huse, E., & Flor, H. (1999). Does use of a myoelectric prosthesis prevent cortical reorganization and phantom limb pain? *Nature Neuroscience, 2*(6), 501–502.
13. Resnik, L. J., Borgia, M. L., Acluche, F., Cancio, J. M., Latlief, G., & Sasson, N. (2018). How do the outcomes of the DEKA Arm compare to conventional prostheses? *PLoS One, 13*(1), e0191326.
14. Clement, R. G., Bugler, K. E., & Oliver, C. W. (2011). Bionic prosthetic hands: A review of present technology and future aspirations. *The Surgeon, 9*(6), 336–340.
15. Abd, M. A., & Engeberg, E. D. (2024). Multichannel sensorimotor integration with a dexterous artificial hand. *Robotics, 13*(7), 97.
16. Sturma, A., Boesendorfer, A., Gstoettner, C., Baumgartner, B., Salminger, S., Farina, D., et al. (2024). Long-term functional and clinical outcome of combined targeted muscle reinnervation and osseointegration for functional bionic reconstruction in transhumeral amputees: A case series. *Journal of Rehabilitation Medicine, 56*, 34141.

17. Fifer, M. S., Hotson, G., Wester, B. A., McMullen, D. P., Wang, Y., Johannes, M. S., et al. (2013). Simultaneous neural control of simple reaching and grasping with the modular prosthetic limb using intracranial EEG. *IEEE Transactions on Neural Systems and Rehabilitation Engineering, 22*(3), 695–705.
18. Cipriani, C., Controzzi, M., & Carrozza, M. C. (2011). The SmartHand transradial prosthesis. *Journal of Neuroengineering and Rehabilitation, 8*(1), 29.
19. Finn, A. P., Grewal, D. S., & Vajzovic, L. (2018). Argus II retinal prosthesis system: A review of patient selection criteria, surgical considerations, and post-operative outcomes. *Clinical Ophthalmology, 12*, 1089–1097.
20. Johansson, R. S., & Flanagan, J. R. (2009). Coding and use of tactile signals from the fingertips in object manipulation tasks. *Nature Reviews Neuroscience, 10*(5), 345–359.
21. Pacchierotti, C., Sinclair, S., Solazzi, M., Frisoli, A., Hayward, V., & Prattichizzo, D. (2017). Wearable haptic systems for the fingertip and the hand: Taxonomy, review, and perspectives. *IEEE Transactions on Haptics, 10*(4), 580–600.
22. El Rassi, I., & El Rassi, J. M. (2020). A review of haptic feedback in tele-operated robotic surgery. *Journal of Medical Engineering & Technology, 44*(5), 247–254.
23. Slater, M., & Sanchez-Vives, M. V. (2016). Enhancing our lives with immersive virtual reality. *Frontiers in Robotics and AI, 3*, 74.

Ethical, Technical, and Regulatory Challenges

5

The clinical promise of AI-powered haptic technology examined in Chaps. 2–4 can only be responsibly realized if the ethical, technical, and regulatory dimensions of its deployment are rigorously addressed. This chapter confronts the most consequential challenges facing AI-haptic healthcare systems: the protection of sensitive biometric and clinical data; the ethical obligations clinicians and developers assume when AI mediates medical decisions; the detection and mitigation of algorithmic bias and opacity; the reliability and safety engineering required of haptic hardware; the navigation of complex international regulatory pathways; the practical barriers to clinical integration; and the equity imperatives that determine whether these technologies reach all patients or deepen existing disparities. Together these themes constitute the responsible innovation agenda that must accompany every stage of AI-haptic system design, deployment, and post-market stewardship.

5.1 Data Privacy and Security in AI Healthcare

AI-haptic systems are uniquely sensitive from a data privacy perspective. Unlike conventional medical devices that generate discrete measurements, AI-haptic systems produce continuous, high-frequency biometric streams including force application patterns, limb trajectory kinematics, EMG signals, and grip dynamics, which are individually identifiable and clinically revealing. These streams encode information about neurological function, physical capacity, and disease progression that patients may reasonably expect to remain private, yet which must flow continuously between sensors, edge processors, cloud AI servers, and electronic health record systems to deliver their clinical benefit [1, 2]. Figure 5.1 illustrates risk vectors from each data source and the corresponding regulatory and technical countermeasures.

R. Thanki, *AI Role in Haptic Healthcare*, Synthesis Lectures on Biomedical Engineering, https://doi.org/10.1007/978-3-032-24907-4_5

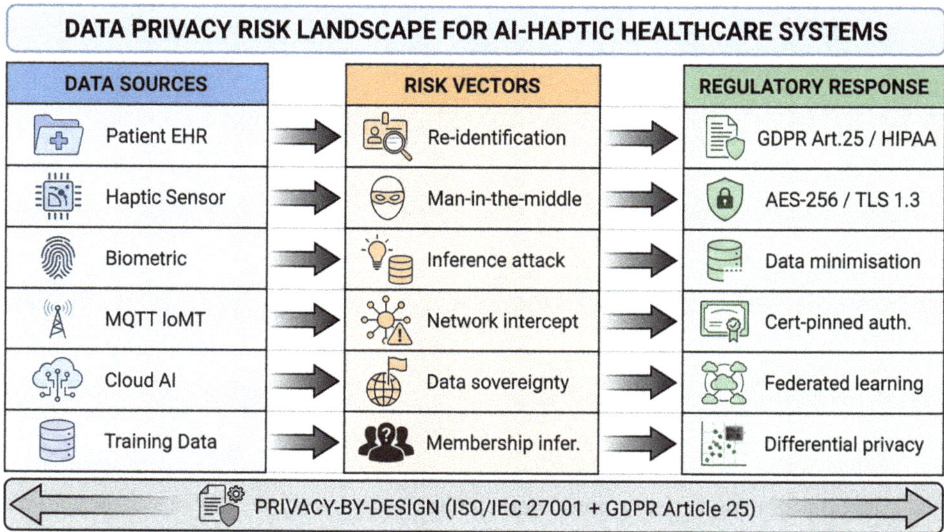

Fig. 5.1 Data privacy risk landscape for AI-haptic healthcare systems

Table 5.1 provides a comparative overview of major privacy and data protection regulations that apply to AI-haptic healthcare systems across different countries and regions. Each row describes a regulation, the jurisdiction where it applies, its scope (whose data or what type of data is covered), and the key legal and technical requirements that organisations must follow to deploy AI-haptic technology in clinical settings.

5.1.1 Privacy Risk Taxonomy for AI-Haptic Systems

Four classes of privacy risk are particularly salient for AI-haptic healthcare systems. Re-identification risk arises when seemingly anonymized haptic movement data is combined with publicly available information. Gait signatures, for example, have been demonstrated to re-identify individuals from anonymous motion capture datasets with over 90% accuracy [2]. Inference attack risk occurs when AI models trained on haptic interaction data inadvertently reveal sensitive clinical information not deliberately collected, for example, grip tremor patterns leaking Parkinson's disease status. Data sovereignty risk arises when haptic data is transmitted to cloud servers in foreign jurisdictions, potentially subject to different legal protections than the patient's country of residence [3]. IoMT interception risk emerges from the wireless transmission paths (MQTT over 5G, Bluetooth Low Energy) connecting wearable haptic sensors to processing infrastructure, which present attack surfaces for man-in-the-middle and replay attacks.

Table 5.1 Privacy and data protection regulations applicable to AI-haptic healthcare systems

Regulation	Jurisdiction	Scope	Key obligations for AI-haptic systems
GDPR (2018)	European Union	Personal data of EU residents	Lawful basis for processing; data minimization; right to erasure; DPIA for high-risk AI; Article 25 privacy-by-design
HIPAA (1996/ updates)	United States	Protected health information (PHI)	PHI encryption; BAAs with AI vendors; minimum necessary standard; audit controls; breach notification
EU AI Act (2024)	European Union	AI systems by risk class	High-risk classification for diagnostic AI; conformity assessment; transparency; human oversight mandate
PDPB/DPDP Act	India	Digital personal data	Consent-based processing; data localization options; health data as sensitive category
PIPL (2021)	China	Personal information of Chinese citizens	Separate consent for sensitive health data; cross-border transfer restrictions; security assessments
MDR 2017/745	European Union	Medical devices (Class I–III)	Post-market surveillance; PMCF; UDI traceability; clinical evidence requirements for SaMD
FDA SaMD guidance	United States	Software as medical device	Predetermined change control plans; real-world performance monitoring; AI/ML action plan

5.1.2 Technical Privacy Controls

Privacy-by-design mandated by GDPR Article 25 and operationalized in ISO/IEC 27701 requires that privacy protections be embedded in system architecture from the outset rather than retrofitted. For AI-haptic systems, this translates to several concrete technical requirements [3]. End-to-end encryption (AES-256 for data at rest, TLS 1.3 for data in transit) protects haptic sensor streams throughout the processing pipeline. Differential privacy, adding mathematically calibrated noise to haptic training datasets, limits the ability of membership inference attacks to determine whether a specific patient's data was included in model training [4]. Federated learning addresses data sovereignty by keeping raw patient data on hospital-controlled edge infrastructure, transmitting only gradient updates to the central AI server. Secure multi-party computation enables multiple hospitals to jointly train AI models on combined datasets without any party observing another's raw data, a particularly valuable technique for rare condition datasets.

Minimum data collection, the principle that only data strictly necessary for the clinical function should be acquired, requires re-evaluation as AI capabilities expand. An AI-haptic system that continuously records full kinematic trajectories when only force magnitude is needed for its clinical function violates the data minimization principle. Data flow mapping, conducted as part of the mandatory Data Protection Impact Assessment (DPIA) under GDPR Article 35, should identify each data element collected, its necessity, its storage location, and its retention period [3].

5.2   Ethical Issues in AI-Assisted Medical Decisions

When AI systems mediate clinical decision-making recommending procedures, alerting surgeons to tissue danger, or guiding rehabilitation intensity, they interpose a technological agent between clinician judgement and patient outcome. This interposition raises profound ethical questions that neither biomedical ethics nor AI ethics alone is sufficient to address questions about consent, responsibility, trust, dependency, and the character of the clinical relationship itself [5, 6].

Figure 5.2 illustrates an ethical decision framework for an AI-haptic medical system that integrates beneficence, non-maleficence, autonomy, justice, explicability, and accountability. Table 5.2 is intended to summarize and compare the main privacy and data protection regulations that apply to AI-haptic healthcare systems. These systems use artificial intelligence and haptic (touch-based) technology to assist with medical decisions, such as surgery or rehabilitation.

5.2.1   Informed Consent in AI-Mediated Haptic Care

The doctrine of informed consent requires that patients understand the nature of their treatment and voluntarily agree to it. When AI systems generate haptic guidance that directly influences a surgical procedure or rehabilitation exercise, the patient's right to understand

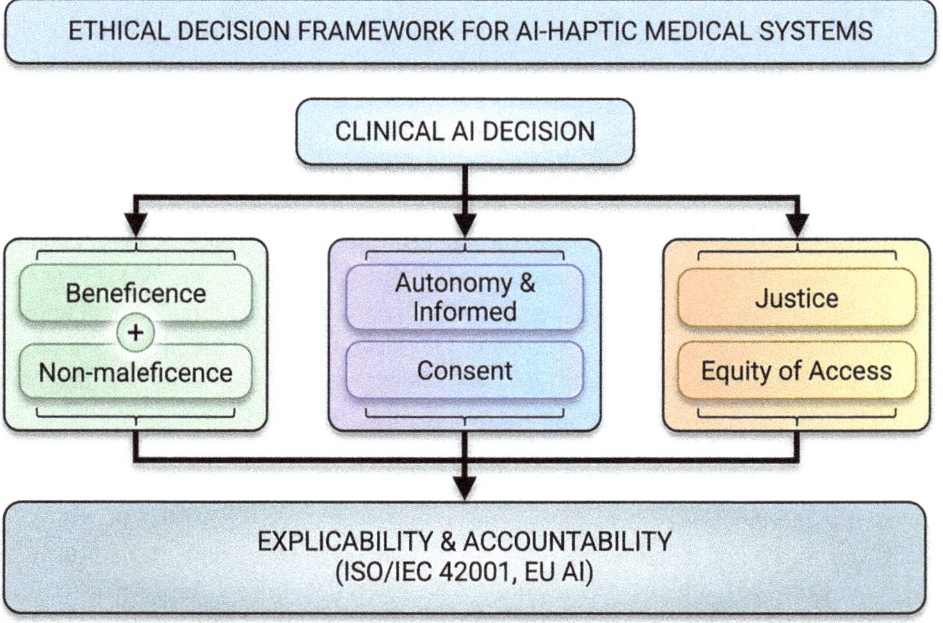

Fig. 5.2 Ethical decision framework for AI-haptic medical systems

Table 5.2 Ethical principles matrix for AI-haptic healthcare systems

Principle	Source framework	AI-haptic system requirement	Implementation strategy
Beneficence	Belmont report	System must demonstrably improve clinical outcomes	Prospective RCTs; outcome monitoring; benefit-risk assessment
Non-maleficence	Beauchamp and Childress	No preventable harm from AI errors or device failure	Fault detection; force limits; fail-safe degradation; FMEA
Autonomy	UNESCO AI ethics	Patients informed about AI role in their care	Informed consent processes; opt-out mechanisms; human override
Justice	WHO AI ethics	Equitable access across demographic groups	Bias audits; affordability planning; multilingual interfaces
Explicability	EU AI Act	AI decisions explainable to clinical users	XAI dashboards; Grad-CAM overlays; confidence-encoded haptics
Accountability	ISO/IEC 42001	Clear responsibility for AI-driven outcomes	Audit trails; version control; post-market surveillance plans
Sustainability	UN SDGs	Long-term responsible deployment	Open standards; modular upgrades; e-waste planning

the role of AI in their care is implicated [2]. Practically, this requires consent forms and processes that describe AI involvement in accessible language not merely noting that a 'computer-assisted' device is used but explaining that an AI system will classify their tissue in real time and modulate surgical forces accordingly, and that the surgeon always retains override authority. Patients must also be informed of the AI system's known performance limitations, including accuracy rates on populations like themselves and the possibility of AI errors. Opt-out mechanisms—the ability for a patient to request that AI guidance features be deactivated while the basic robotic or haptic device continues to function— are both ethically important and technically challenging to implement, requiring system architectures that separate AI augmentation from core device functionality [5].

5.2.2   Responsibility and Liability Attribution

When an AI-haptic system contributes to an adverse patient outcome, a misclassified tissue leading to inadvertent vessel injury, or a rehabilitation device applying excessive force, the attribution of clinical and legal responsibility is deeply contested. The traditional malpractice framework assigns responsibility to the treating clinician; yet where an AI system overrides or constrains clinician action, the device manufacturer and AI developer share at least partial causal responsibility for the outcome [7].

The EU AI Act (2024) addresses this in part by requiring that high-risk AI systems including those used in surgical and rehabilitation contexts maintain comprehensive audit trails enabling post-incident reconstruction of the AI system's inputs, outputs, and confidence levels at every moment of the procedure [3]. This requirement has significant implications for AI-haptic system design: every AI inference, every haptic command generated, and every surgeon override must be logged with timestamps to microsecond precision, creating an irrefutable record of the AI's contribution to the clinical event. Liability frameworks must evolve in parallel, with insurance products, clinical governance policies, and professional standards addressing the shared responsibility model that AI-mediated clinical care necessitates.

5.2.3 Clinical Dependency and Deskilling

A subtle but consequential ethical risk of AI-haptic systems is the potential for clinicians to deskilling the atrophy of manual surgical or diagnostic skills that results from habitual reliance on AI assistance [8]. If surgeons trained exclusively in AI-haptic-assisted environments lack the tactile competence to operate safely when the AI system fails or is unavailable— as may occur in emergency contexts, resource-limited settings, or during system downtime— patient safety is compromised. Training curricula must explicitly include AI-off scenarios, and professional standards bodies should establish minimum manual competency requirements that AI-assisted practice must supplement, not replace.

5.3 Bias and Transparency in AI Algorithms

Algorithmic bias in clinical AI systems is not a theoretical concern: a landmark study demonstrated that a widely used commercial healthcare algorithm systematically underestimated the health needs of Black patients compared to equally sick White patients, because it used healthcare costs as a proxy for health needs reflecting historical patterns of unequal access rather than underlying disease burden [9]. AI-haptic systems face structurally analogous bias risks arising from unrepresentative training data, biased labelling processes, and the deployment of models trained on one patient population to serve another.

5.3.1 Sources of Bias in AI-Haptic Systems

Training data representation bias is the most pervasive risk. Haptic surgical datasets are predominantly collected at high-volume academic medical centres in North America and Western Europe, skewing models toward patients with body compositions, tissue properties, and disease presentations typical of those populations [9]. AI tissue classification models trained on such datasets may perform significantly worse for patients with higher BMI, different skin tones affecting optical tissue properties, or disease presentations prevalent in other geographic regions. Measurement bias arises from sensor calibration differences across device instances and clinical sites: a model trained on force measurements from one sensor manufacturer may produce systematically biased predictions when deployed on a device with a different sensor with different noise characteristics.

Label bias emerges when the ground truth annotations used to train AI models reflect the biases of the annotating clinicians. In haptic surgical training datasets, tissue labels assigned by expert surgeons encode their clinical experience and perceptual expectations which may themselves reflect biased training environments. Automation biases the tendency of clinicians to over-trust and under-question AI outputs can amplify the clinical impact of algorithmic bias: if a surgeon trusts an AI tissue classification alert without independent verification, a biased classification directly influences procedural decisions [8]. Table 5.3 catalogues the major bias types affecting AI-haptic systems from historical and representation bias to automation and feedback loop bias detailing their origins, clinical risks, and recommended mitigation strategies. Figure 5.3 maps the full AI bias lifecycle in healthcare haptic systems, tracing how bias enters at data collection, propagates through training, and manifests during deployment, with the corresponding mitigation tools and XAI transparency layer overlaid at each stage.

5.3.2 Transparency and Explainability Requirements

The EU AI Act classifies AI systems used in surgical and rehabilitation medical devices as high-risk, mandating that they provide explanations of their decisions in a manner meaningful to qualified users [3]. ISO/IEC 42001:2023 further operationalizes this as a

Table 5.3 Bias types in AI-haptic systems

Bias type	Origin	Clinical risk	Mitigation strategy
Historical bias	Biased training labels	Incorrect tissue classification	Diverse annotator panels; label audit; prospective re-labelling
Representation bias	Non-diverse datasets	Poor performance on under-represented demographics	Stratified data collection; federated learning across sites
Measurement bias	Sensor calibration drift	Force rendering errors accumulating over time	Regular recalibration schedules; drift-detection algorithms
Aggregation bias	Population-averaged models	Fails individual patient edge cases	Personalized fine-tuning; uncertainty quantification
Automation bias	Over-trust in AI alerts	Surgeon ignores valid clinical judgement	Training protocols; confidence thresholds displayed to user
Feedback loop bias	AI learns from its own outputs	Performance degradation amplifies over time	Ground truth validation; independent test set monitoring
Deployment bias	Train-test distribution shift	Model degrades in new hospital context	Domain adaptation; PMCF monitoring; performance drift alerts

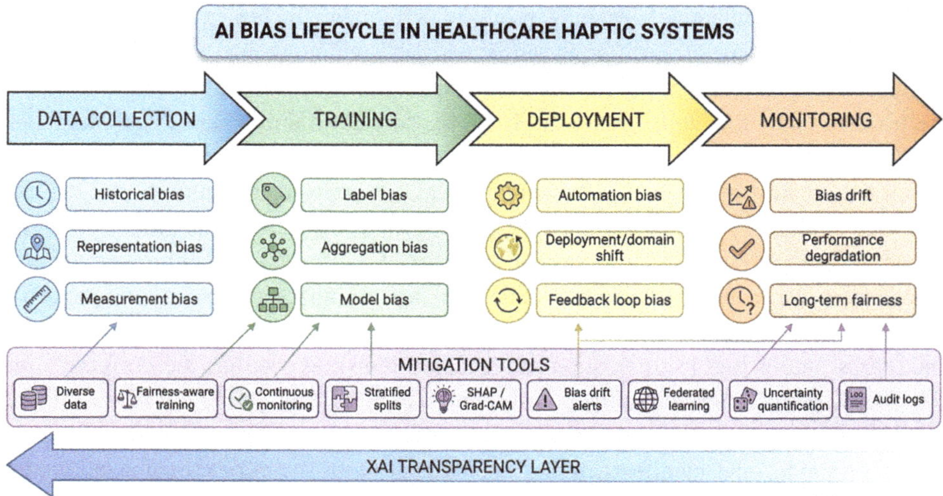

Fig. 5.3 AI bias lifecycle in healthcare haptic systems

management system requirement. In the haptic domain, transparency must be expressed through the haptic modality itself, not merely through a separate visual display that adds to cognitive load because surgeons' hands and attention are already engaged during procedures.

Explainable AI (XAI) techniques applicable to AI-haptic systems include: SHAP (SHapley Additive exPlanations) values that quantify each sensor feature's contribution to a tissue classification decision; Grad-CAM applied to the concurrent video feed to highlight the anatomical region driving the AI alert; and confidence-encoded haptic rendering in which the intensity or pattern of the haptic cue encodes the model's classification confidence [10]. A high-confidence vessel proximity alert might be rendered as a sharp, strong force impulse; a low-confidence advisory might be rendered as a gentle, slow vibrotactile pattern communicating not merely the alert but the AI's certainty, allowing the surgeon to calibrate their response appropriately.

5.4 Reliability and Safety of Haptic Devices

Haptic medical devices that apply forces to the human body whether in surgery, rehabilitation, or prosthetic control are safety-critical systems in the formal engineering sense: their failure modes can directly injure patients. Unlike software-only clinical decision support tools, where an incorrect recommendation can be overridden before action, a haptic device that delivers an excessive force impulse to a surgical instrument or rehabilitation orthosis causes immediate physical harm [11, 12]. This reality demands safety engineering rigor equivalent to Class IIb and III medical device standards, applied to both hardware and the AI software components that generate haptic commands.

5.4.1 Failure Mode Analysis and Safety Architecture

ISO 14971:2019 risk management mandates systematic identification of all hazardous situations causes, harms, and probabilities through techniques including Failure Mode and Effects Analysis (FMEA) and Fault Tree Analysis (FTA) [11]. For AI-haptic systems, hazard identification must extend beyond hardware failures (actuator stall, sensor disconnection) to include AI failure modes: out-of-distribution inputs causing misclassification; adversarial sensor noise triggering incorrect haptic commands; and model performance degradation due to distributional shift after deployment.

Safety architecture for AI-haptic systems follows the principle of defence-in-depth: multiple independent safety layers, each capable of preventing harm if upstream layers fail [13] This layered approach ensures that no single point of failure including AI model failure can cause patient injury. Figure 5.4 presents the haptic device safety assurance framework across all three lifecycle phases such as design, verification, and validation, and post-market together with the applicable standards at each stage. Table 5.4 details the different principal standards governing AI-haptic medical device safety, from ISO 14971 risk management and IEC 62304 software lifecycle to ISO/IEC 42001 AI management systems.

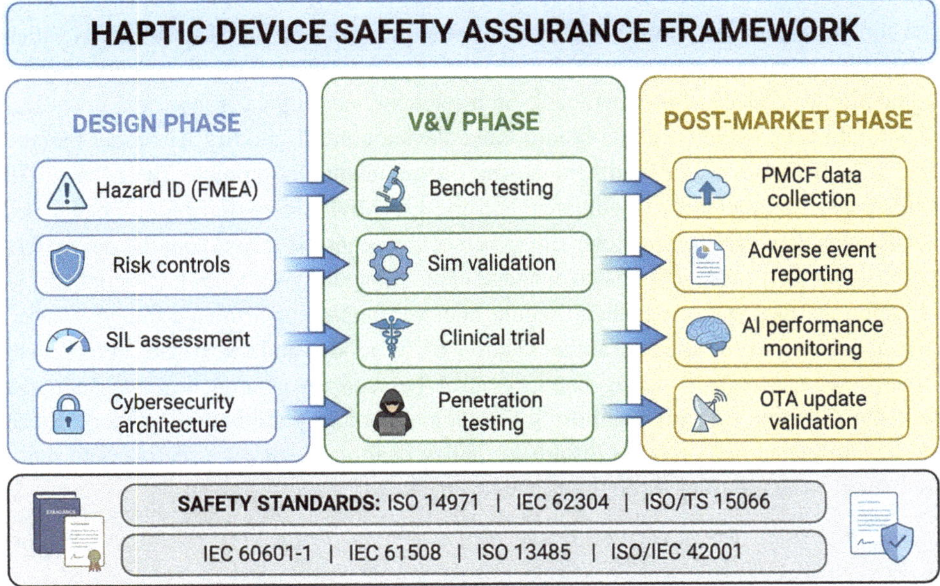

Fig. 5.4 Haptic device safety assurance framework

Table 5.4 Safety and quality standards applicable to AI-haptic medical devices

Standard	Domain	Applicability	Key requirements for haptic AI systems
ISO 14971:2019	Risk management	All medical devices	Hazard identification (FMEA/FTA); risk control; residual risk evaluation
IEC 62304:2006 + A1	Software lifecycle	SaMD components	Class B/C software processes; change management; anomaly resolution
IEC 60601–1	Electrical safety	Active medical devices	Basic safety and essential performance; max contact current limits
ISO/TS 15066:2016	Collaborative robotics	Robotic haptic devices	Biomechanical pain thresholds; power/force limiting; speed monitoring
IEC 61508	Functional safety	Safety-critical control	SIL-1 to SIL-3 classification; probability of failure on demand
ISO 13485:2016	Quality management	Medical device QMS	Design controls; CAPA; supplier qualification; post-market surveillance
ISO/IEC 42001:2023	AI management	AI system governance	AI risk management; transparency; monitoring; human oversight

5.4.2 Cybersecurity as a Patient Safety Requirement

The connectivity of AI-haptic systems to hospital networks, cloud AI servers, and patient monitoring infrastructure creates cybersecurity attack surfaces with direct patient safety implications. A successful cyberattack on a teleoperated surgical robot or a networked rehabilitation exoskeleton could compromise device control, modify AI model parameters, or inject false sensor readings causing dangerous haptic outputs. The FDA's 2023 medical device cybersecurity guidance and the EU MDR's essential requirements both mandate that manufacturers implement cybersecurity controls throughout the device lifecycle including post-market patch management. Mandatory cybersecurity controls for AI-haptic medical systems include: secure boot verification of firmware integrity before each activation; cryptographic authentication of AI model updates before deployment; network segmentation isolating haptic control buses from general hospital networks; intrusion detection systems monitoring for anomalous data patterns indicative of attack; and a coordinated vulnerability disclosure policy enabling security researchers to report discovered vulnerabilities through official channels [14].

5.4.3 Verification, Validation, and Testing

IEC 62304 classifies medical device software by the severity of harm its failure could cause: Class A (no injury), Class B (non-serious injury), and Class C (serious injury or death) [14]. AI inference software generating force commands in a surgical haptic system would typically be classified Class C, requiring the most rigorous software development lifecycle including unit testing, integration testing, system testing, and regression testing after every model update. Testing must cover not only nominal operation but edge cases, boundary conditions, and out-of-distribution inputs that the system may encounter in clinical use.

5.5   Regulatory Frameworks for AI Medical Technologies

The regulatory landscape for AI medical technologies is undergoing its most significant transformation in decades, driven by the convergence of AI-specific regulation (EU AI Act), evolving medical device frameworks (EU MDR, FDA SaMD guidance), and the emergence of international AI governance standards (ISO/IEC 42001). AI-haptic devices that combine physical actuation with AI-driven decision-making fall at the intersection of multiple regulatory frameworks simultaneously, requiring manufacturers to satisfy the requirements of all applicable frameworks, a multi-dimensional compliance challenge without clear precedent [15, 16].

5.5.1   EU Medical Device Regulation (MDR 2017/745)

Under EU MDR 2017/745, AI-haptic devices are classified based on the risk they pose to patients. A robotic surgical system with active force feedback would typically be classified Class IIb (active therapeutic device with risk of injury) or Class III (implantable or life-supporting) [15]. Class IIb and III devices require conformity assessment by a notified body, an independent third-party organisation authorized by an EU member state which reviews the technical documentation, clinical evaluation, and quality management system before CE marking is granted. The clinical evaluation must include a clinical investigation (prospective study) for Class III devices unless an equivalence claim can be substantiated for an existing, already-certified device.

A critical requirement introduced by MDR and directly relevant to AI-haptic systems is the Post-Market Clinical Follow-up (PMCF) obligation: manufacturers must continuously collect real-world clinical data from deployed devices and update their clinical evidence with reference to a pre-specified PMCF plan. For AI models that improve through post-deployment learning, changes must be evaluated against a Predetermined Change Control Plan (PCCP) specifying the boundaries of allowable AI update without triggering full re-certification [15].

5.5.2   FDA Software as a Medical Device (SaMD) Framework

The FDA's AI/ML Action Plan (2021) and subsequent guidance documents establish a risk-stratified framework for AI-based SaMD, where risk classification depends on the significance of the AI system's function (treating versus informing) and the state of the healthcare situation (critical versus non-critical) [16]. AI systems that directly drive surgical haptic force outputs rather than merely advising the surgeon would be classified at the highest risk tier, requiring Premarket Approval (PMA) with clinical evidence demonstrating safety and effectiveness. This framework explicitly acknowledges the iteratively improving nature of ML-based medical devices while maintaining regulatory oversight of meaningful changes.

Figure 5.5 maps the complete regulatory pathway for AI-haptic medical devices across EU MDR and FDA frameworks by risk class, highlighting where PCCP requirements apply to AI/ML components. Table 5.5 provides a comparative overview of all major international regulatory pathways from EU MDR and FDA PMA to Germany's DiGA pathway and India's CDSCO framework with the key requirements for each jurisdiction.

5.5.3   ISO/IEC 42001 AI Management System Standard

ISO/IEC 42001:2023, the first international standard for AI management systems provides an organisational governance framework that complements product-level regulatory requirements [7]. It requires organisations developing or deploying AI in healthcare to establish policies, processes, and controls governing AI risk assessment, transparency,

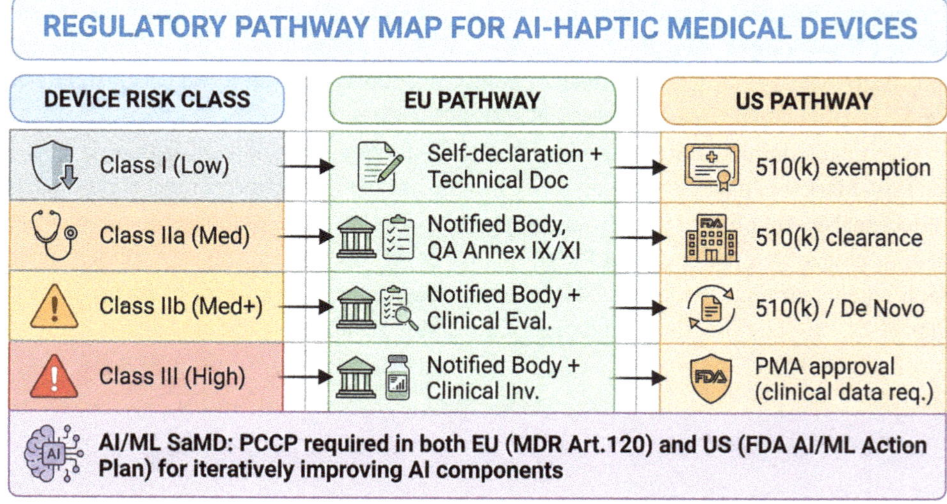

Fig. 5.5 Regulatory pathway map for AI-haptic medical devices

Table 5.5 International regulatory pathways for AI-haptic medical devices

Framework	Jurisdiction	Device class	Key pathway requirements
EU MDR 2017/745	European Union	Class IIa–III	Technical documentation; clinical evaluation; notified body QA; EUDAMED registration; PMCF
FDA 510(k)	United States	Class II (moderate risk)	Substantial equivalence to predicate; performance testing; labelling; cybersecurity documentation
FDA PMA	United States	Class III (high risk)	Valid scientific evidence of safety/ effectiveness; clinical study data; manufacturing inspection
FDA AI/ML action plan	United States	AI-based SaMD	PCCP; algorithm change protocol; real-world performance monitoring plan
DiGA pathway	Germany	Digital health apps	Fast-track 12-week review; evidence of positive care effect; interoperability; data security
MHRA UK CA	United Kingdom	Post-Brexit MDR	Software qualification; clinical evaluation; UKCA marking; approved body assessment
CDSCO	India	Medical devices	Class B–D; clinical investigation waiver options; manufacturing site registration

human oversight, and continuous improvement. For AI-haptic device manufacturers, implementing ISO/IEC 42001 provides a structured foundation for demonstrating regulatory compliance across multiple jurisdictions, because its requirements map closely to the AI governance provisions of the EU AI Act, FDA SaMD guidance, and emerging national AI regulations in India, China, and the UK.

5.6   Integration Challenges in Clinical Environments

The transition forms a promising research prototype to a routinely deployed clinical tool, which is one of the most challenging phases in medical technology development. AI-haptic systems face integration barriers that span technical infrastructure, organisational processes, clinical culture, and economic constraints barriers that are distinct from and often more formidable than the technical challenges of creating the device itself.

5.6.1   Technical Integration Barriers

Interoperability with legacy health information systems is the most pervasive technical integration challenge. Most hospital electronic health records (EHRs) in active use were developed before HL7 FHIR R4 became the interoperability standard; connecting AI-haptic systems to these systems requires bespoke middleware adapters, custom data mapping, and negotiation with EHR vendors over API access. Network infrastructure in older hospital buildings frequently lacks the bandwidth, latency, and reliability required to support AI-haptic real-time data flows; 5G or dedicated Wi-Fi 6 infrastructure upgrades may be necessary before deployment, adding capital costs not typically included in device acquisition budgets.

Sensor calibration and maintenance represent ongoing operational integration challenges. Haptic device sensors drift over time; AI models trained on well-calibrated sensor data produce degraded outputs when deployed on sensors that have drifted. Automated self-calibration routines, predictive maintenance models that flag sensor degradation before it affects clinical performance, and clear maintenance protocols integrated with hospital biomedical engineering schedules are all necessary components of a sustainable AI-haptic deployment [17].

5.6.2 Organisational and Human Integration Challenges

Clinician trust is the most critical non-technical integration requirement. A technically excellent AI-haptic system that clinician's distrust will be actively circumvented alerts silenced, AI features disabled, or devices abandoned in favour of familiar manual techniques [8]. Trust must be earned through transparent communication of performance data, clinical involvement in device co-design, and progressive deployment strategies that allow clinicians to gain confidence in AI-haptic capabilities before relying on them for complex procedures. Clinical champions, respected senior clinicians who advocate for technology within their peer group, are one of the most consistently effective strategies for accelerating trust and adoption. Human factors engineering involving clinicians, nurses, and patients as co-designers from the earliest prototype stage is the most reliable method for achieving workflow-compatible integration.

Figure 5.6 presents a sociotechnical map of the clinical integration challenges facing AI-haptic systems, organizing barriers across three layers, technical, organisational, and human, and identifying a co-design and phased rollout strategy for each.

Table 5.6 structures these integration challenges by domain, specifying the barriers, affected stakeholders, and evidence-based mitigation approaches.

5.7 Cost, Accessibility, and Healthcare Equity

The clinical benefits demonstrated for AI-haptic systems in Chaps. 3 and 4 improved surgical precision, accelerated rehabilitation, restored prosthetic sensation are overwhelmingly documented in high-income hospital settings in North America, Western Europe, and East Asia. If the economic and infrastructural barriers to AI-haptic deployment remain unaddressed, these technologies risk amplifying existing health disparities rather than reducing them: high-income patients receive AI-enhanced surgical care while low-income patients continue to receive standard-of-care surgery with greater complication rates [5, 18].

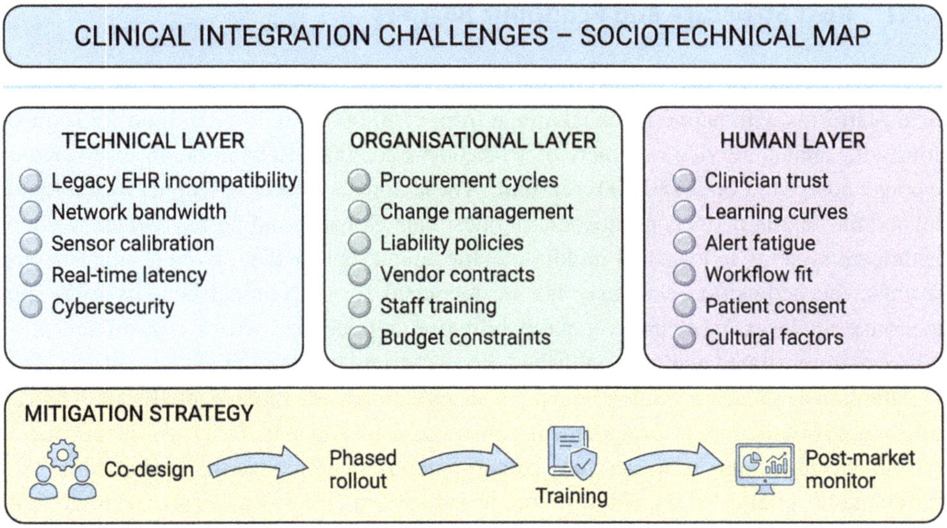

CLINICAL INTEGRATION CHALLENGES – SOCIOTECHNICAL MAP

TECHNICAL LAYER
- Legacy EHR incompatibility
- Network bandwidth
- Sensor calibration
- Real-time latency
- Cybersecurity

ORGANISATIONAL LAYER
- Procurement cycles
- Change management
- Liability policies
- Vendor contracts
- Staff training
- Budget constraints

HUMAN LAYER
- Clinician trust
- Learning curves
- Alert fatigue
- Workflow fit
- Patient consent
- Cultural factors

MITIGATION STRATEGY

Fig. 5.6 Clinical integration challenges

Table 5.6 AI-haptic clinical integration challenges and mitigation approaches

Challenge domain	Specific barrier	Affected stakeholder	Mitigation approach
Interoperability	Legacy EHR incompatibility	Hospital IT, clinicians	HL7 FHIR R4 APIs; IHE integration profiles; middleware adapters
Workflow disruption	Procedure time increase	Surgeons, OR staff	Co-design with end users; phased rollout; simulation training
Calibration and maintenance	Sensor drift over time	Biomedical engineering	Automated self-calibration; predictive maintenance AI; OTA firmware
Staff training	Learning curve for new interfaces	All clinical users	Simulation-based training; competency assessment; refresher modules
Infrastructure	Insufficient network bandwidth	Hospital IT	5G/Wi-Fi 6 upgrade; edge computing offload; QoS prioritization
Vendor lock-in	Proprietary data formats	Procurement, IT	Open API requirements in procurement; data portability clauses
Change management	Clinician resistance to AI	Clinicians, management	Clinical champions; evidence-based value demonstrations; co-design

5.7.1 Cost Structure and Economic Barriers

The cost of AI-haptic systems in clinical-grade configurations is substantial. Robotic surgical platforms with haptic feedback range from €500,000 to over €2 million for acquisition, with annual service contracts of €100,000–€200,000. Rehabilitation exoskeletons average cost €40,000–€150,000 per unit. These figures place AI-haptic technologies beyond the capital budgets of most district hospitals globally, and far beyond the reach of healthcare systems in low- and middle-income countries (LMICs). Even in high-income settings, the acquisition cost may not be recouped by the clinical benefits in health-economic analyses, particularly for rehabilitation applications where cost-effectiveness must be demonstrated against established physiotherapy interventions.

Alternative financing models, device-as-a-service leasing, shared platforms between multiple hospitals, public procurement consortia, and outcomes-based payment models that tie device revenue to measurable patient outcomes can reduce the capital barrier for individual hospitals [18]. Health technology assessment (HTA) bodies (NICE in the UK, IQWiG in Germany, HAS in France) must develop AI-specific evaluation frameworks that capture long-term outcomes, quality-adjusted life year improvements, and system-level cost savings from reduced complication rates and shorter hospital stays.

5.7.2 Technology Design for Global Health Equity

Healthcare equity demands that AI-haptic technologies be designed from the outset for deployment across a spectrum of healthcare settings not engineered for tertiary academic medical centres and then 'simplified' for other contexts as an afterthought. Design-for-equity principles include modularity (enabling core haptic functionality to be deployed without the full suite of AI features in resource-constrained settings); offline capability (edge AI inference that functions without continuous internet connectivity); open-source software components (reducing per-unit software licensing costs); and multilingual, culturally adapted user interfaces [18]. The clinical validation evidence base for AI-haptic technologies is itself geographically inequitable: virtually all published clinical trials have been conducted in Europe, North America, and East Asia. Regulatory agencies in LMICs cannot reasonably approve devices based on evidence drawn from patient populations that do not represent their citizens [19]. International research collaboration programmes, funded by WHO, the Wellcome Trust, and bilateral government partnerships are needed to build the multi-site clinical evidence base that supports regulatory approval and clinical confidence across diverse global healthcare systems.

5.7.3   Policy Levers for Equitable AI-Haptic Access

Several policy mechanisms can accelerate equitable access to AI-haptic healthcare technologies. Regulatory fast-track pathways analogous to Germany's DiGA pathway for digital health apps could be established specifically for AI-haptic devices that demonstrate measurable patient benefit, reducing the time and cost of market authorisations for devices targeting underserved patient populations [15]. Compulsory technology transfer agreements requiring that manufacturers receiving public research funding make their AI models and training data available under open licenses would enable LMIC innovators to build on existing advances rather than duplicating them. Global Health Technology Assessment frameworks, aligned with WHO's model list methodology, should establish universal criteria for AI-haptic HTA that are applicable across income settings and incorporate equity as an explicit evaluation dimension [5].

5.8   Summary

This chapter explores the ethical, technical, and regulatory challenges of AI-powered haptic healthcare systems, emphasizing the need for responsible innovation to ensure privacy, safety, equity, and effective clinical integration. It highlights the importance of robust data privacy measures, ethical considerations in AI-mediated medical decisions, and strategies to mitigate algorithmic bias. The chapter underscores the safety-critical nature of haptic devices, requiring rigorous engineering standards, cybersecurity controls, and comprehensive testing. It also examines the complex regulatory landscape, including compliance with frameworks like the EU MDR, FDA SaMD guidance, and ISO/IEC 42001. Integration challenges such as interoperability, clinician trust, and training are addressed through co-design and phased deployment strategies. Finally, the chapter stresses the need for equitable access to AI-haptic technologies, advocating for design-for-equity principles, alternative financing models, and global collaboration to reduce healthcare disparities.

References

1. Topol, E. J. (2019). High-performance medicine: The convergence of human and artificial intelligence. *Nature Medicine, 25*(1), 44–56.
2. Char, D. S., Shah, N. H., & Magnus, D. (2018). Implementing machine learning in health care—Addressing ethical challenges. *The New England Journal of Medicine, 378*(11), 981.
3. European Parliament. (2024). Regulation (EU) 2024/1689—Artificial Intelligence Act. *Official Journal of the European Union*, L 2024/1689.
4. McMahan, B., Moore, E., Ramage, D., Hampson, S., & y Arcas, B. A. (2017, April). Communication-efficient learning of deep networks from decentralized data. In *Artificial intelligence and statistics* (pp. 1273–1282). PMLR.

5. World Health Organization. (2021). *Ethics and governance of artificial intelligence for health.* WHO Press. https://www.who.int/publications/i/item/9789240029200

6. Jobin, A., Ienca, M., & Vayena, E. (2019). The global landscape of AI ethics guidelines. *Nature Machine Intelligence, 1*(9), 389–399.

7. Taddeo, M., & Floridi, L. (2018). How AI can be a force for good. *Science, 361*(6404), 751–752.

8. Obermeyer, Z., & Emanuel, E. J. (2016). Predicting the future—Big data, machine learning, and clinical medicine. *The New England Journal of Medicine, 375*(13), 1216.

9. Obermeyer, Z., Powers, B., Vogeli, C., & Mullainathan, S. (2019). Dissecting racial bias in an algorithm used to manage the health of populations. *Science, 366*(6464), 447–453.

10. Wachter, S., Mittelstadt, B., & Russell, C. (2017). Counterfactual explanations without opening the black box: Automated decisions and the GDPR. *Harvard Journal of Law & Technology, 31*, 841.

11. International Organization for Standardization. (2019). *ISO 14971:2019—Medical devices— Application of risk management.* ISO.

12. International Organization for Standardization. (2016). *ISO/TS 15066:2016—Robots and robotic devices—Collaborative robots.* ISO.

13. Haddadin, S., & Croft, E. (2016). Physical human–robot interaction. In *Springer handbook of robotics* (pp. 1835–1874). Springer.

14. International Electrotechnical Commission. (2015). *IEC 62304:2006+AMD1:2015—Medical device software—Software life cycle processes.* IEC.

15. European Commission. (2017). Regulation (EU) 2017/745—Medical Device Regulation. *Official Journal of the European Union.*

16. U.S. Food and Drug Administration. (2021). *Artificial intelligence and machine learning (AI/ ML)-based software as a medical device (SaMD) action plan.* FDA.

17. Pacchierotti, C., Sinclair, S., Solazzi, M., Frisoli, A., Hayward, V., & Prattichizzo, D. (2017). Wearable haptic systems for the fingertip and the hand: Taxonomy, review, and perspectives. *IEEE Transactions on Haptics, 10*(4), 580–600.

18. United Nations General Assembly (2015). *Transforming our world: the 2030 Agenda for Sustainable Development.*

19. Abràmoff, M. D., Lavin, P. T., Birch, M., Shah, N., & Folk, J. C. (2018). Pivotal trial of an autonomous AI-based diagnostic system for detection of diabetic retinopathy in primary care offices. *npj Digital Medicine, 1*(1), 39.

Future Trends and Innovations in AI-Driven Haptic Healthcare

6

This concluding chapter looks beyond the technologies deployed and the challenges addressed in Chaps. 2–5 to map the emerging and visionary frontiers of AI-driven haptic healthcare. Seven thematic threads are examined: the near-to-long-term technology landscape of novel haptic interfaces spanning microfluidic skins, neuromorphic chips, and the haptic internet; the convergence of brain–computer interfaces with sensory feedback to restore and augment natural touch; the promise of soft robotics and biomimetic materials for the next generation of prosthetics; the integration of AI-haptic systems within smart hospital digital ecosystems and digital twin architectures; the role of multi-omics personalization in tailoring haptic medicine to individual patients; a structured research and innovation roadmap extending to 2040; and a synthesis vision for the collaborative future of human and machine intelligence in tactile medicine. Throughout, the responsible innovation principles established in Chap. 5 are carried forward as the ethical substrate upon which these futures must be built.

6.1 Emerging Technologies in Haptic Interfaces

The haptic interface technologies that underpin current clinical AI-haptic systems force-feedback robotic arms, vibrotactile wristbands, and electrotactile fingertip stimulators represent the first generation of a rapidly expanding technology landscape. Across materials science, microelectronics, and neuroscience, a convergent set of innovations is approaching clinical readiness that will fundamentally expand the bandwidth, resolution, naturalness, and wearability of haptic human–machine interaction in healthcare [1, 2].

R. Thanki, *AI Role in Haptic Healthcare*, Synthesis Lectures on Biomedical Engineering, https://doi.org/10.1007/978-3-032-24907-4_6

6.1.1   Mid-Air and Touchless Haptic Interfaces

Mid-air ultrasonic haptic displays arrays of focused ultrasound transducers that create tactile sensations on the bare skin without physical contact are among the most clinically promising near-term interface innovations. In operating room contexts, surgeons must maintain sterile fields throughout procedures; any interface requiring physical contact with a control device risks contamination. Mid-air haptic arrays positioned above the scrub table could enable surgeons to adjust robotic parameters, approve AI recommendations, and navigate imaging data through touchless gestural interaction with tactile confirmation, eliminating the need for circulating nurses to handle contamination-prone touchscreens [1]. Current mid-air ultrasonic arrays (Ultrahaptics/Ultraleap) achieve tactile point resolution of approximately 1 cm at forces up to 16 mN sufficient for button-press confirmation but not yet for rich tissue texture rendering, which requires forces of 0.1–1 N and spatial resolution below 2 mm.

6.1.2   Soft Microfluidic and Electronic Skin

Soft microfluidic haptic skins, consisting of flexible silicone substrates embedding arrays of pneumatic microchannels that individually inflate to deliver distributed pressure and thermal stimulation, represent a paradigm shift from the point-contact haptic actuators of current wearable devices toward full-hand, conformally wearable haptic interfaces [3]. These devices can wrap the entire hand in an active tactile surface, rendering spatially distributed contact patterns such as the progressive engagement of finger pads during a grasping movement with spatial resolution approaching the two-point discrimination threshold of the human fingertip (approximately 2–5 mm on the palm). AI control architectures for soft microfluidic skins must solve the high-dimensional actuation problem: coordinating hundreds of individually addressable pneumatic channels to produce coherent tactile patterns requires generative AI models trained on human psychophysical data to map desired perceptual experiences to pneumatic pressure patterns.

Electronic skin (e-skin) technologies, based on nanomaterial sensors such as graphene piezoresistive arrays, carbon nanotube pressure sensors, and silver nanowire strain gauges, enable mechanically flexible tactile sensing at spatial densities approaching the 2500 mechanoreceptors per cm^2 of the human fingertip [4]. Integrated into prosthetic fingers and surgical instruments, e-skin transforms previously tactile-blind interfaces into rich sensing surfaces. AI signal processing pipelines—1D CNNs operating on the dense multi-channel sensor streams—extract clinically meaningful haptic features (tissue stiffness, surface texture, and slip onset) at the rates required for real-time haptic rendering.

Table 6.1 provides a structured comparison of seven emerging haptic interface technologies from mid-air ultrasonic haptics to neuromorphic spike-based systems rating each

Table 6.1 Emerging haptic interface technologies

Technology	Maturity (TRL)	Haptic modality	Clinical promise and current limitations
Mid-air ultrasonic haptics	TRL 5–6	Touchless tactile sensation	Sterile-field OR control; limited force magnitude (<1 N)
Soft microfluidic skin	TRL 4–5	Distributed pressure + thermal	Wearable full-hand haptics; fabrication scalability challenges
Electrostatic skin rendering	TRL 5	Surface friction modulation	Ultra-thin touchscreen haptics; limited 3-D force resolution
Ionotronic hydrogel devices	TRL 3–4	Biomimetic mechanoreception	Implantable bio-compatible haptic skin; long-term stability TBD
Piezoelectric MEMS arrays	TRL 6–7	High-freq. vibrotactile	Tactile texture rendering; limited displacement range
Magnetic levitation haptics	TRL 5–6	6-DOF precision force feedback	Surgical micromanipulation; workspace volume constraints
Neuromorphic spike-based haptics	TRL 3	Event-driven tactile encoding	Ultra-low latency BCI coupling; hardware maturity gap

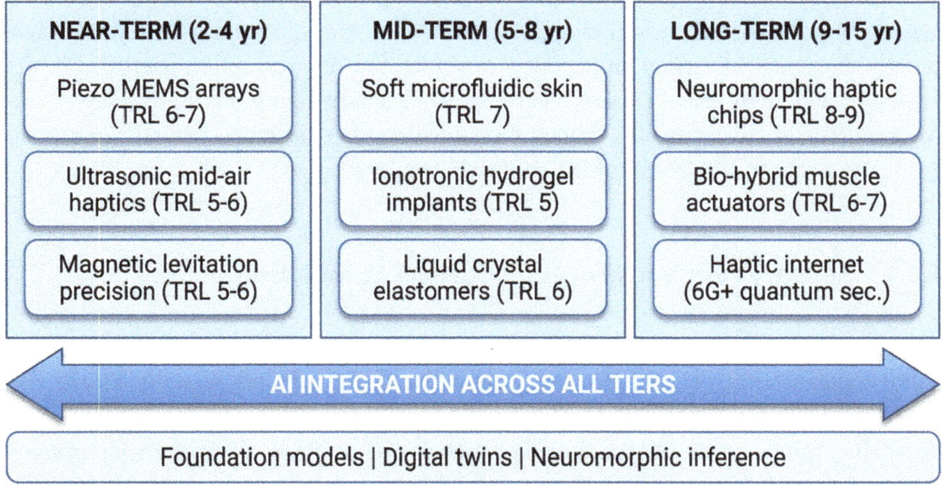

Fig. 6.1 Data privacy risk landscape for AI-haptic healthcare systems

by technology readiness level (TRL), haptic modality, and clinical promise alongside current limitations. Figure 6.1 then maps these technologies across a 2025–2040 timeline, organizing near-term, mid-term, and long-term innovations by maturity tier and showing how AI integration themes foundation models, digital twins, and neuromorphic inference span all tiers.

6.1.3 Neuromorphic Haptic Processing

Neuromorphic computing processing architectures that emulate the event-driven, spike-based computation of biological neural networks offer a revolutionary approach to real-time haptic signal processing. Conventional von Neumann processor architecture introduces latency through memory access bottlenecks that become significant at the microsecond timescales required for high-fidelity haptic rendering. Neuromorphic chips (Intel Loihi 2, IBM NorthPole) process tactile sensor events asynchronously, producing responses in under 100 μs an order of magnitude faster than GPU-accelerated inference while consuming a fraction of the power of conventional edge AI hardware [5]. Neuromorphic haptic encoding architectures, trained through spike-timing-dependent plasticity rules, can learn to represent tactile sensor streams in population codes that directly interface with peripheral nerve stimulation patterns for BCI-haptic applications.

6.2 Brain–Computer Interfaces and Sensory Feedback

Brain–computer interfaces (BCIs) that restore somatosensory feedback represent perhaps the most transformative frontier in AI-haptic healthcare: the prospect of replacing the lost sense of touch not with an artificial device that approximates natural sensation, but by directly engaging the neural architecture of somatosensory perception itself [6, 7]. The convergence of high-density neural recording, AI decoding algorithms, and precision neural stimulation is advancing this vision from laboratory demonstration toward clinical reality at a pace that would have seemed implausible a decade ago.

6.2.1 Sensory Feedback Through Cortical Stimulation

Intracortical microstimulation (ICMS) of primary somatosensory cortex (S1) using chronically implanted microelectrode arrays can evoke tactile percepts spatially localized to specific body regions through the cortical body map (homunculus) [8]. Landmark work by Bensmaia, Miller, and colleagues demonstrated that artificial S1 stimulation patterns encoding contact location, pressure magnitude, and flutter frequency could be distinguished by non-human primates at performance levels comparable to natural touch. In human clinical trials (Brain Gate consortium), participants with tetraplegia receiving ICMS-based sensory feedback through bidirectional BCI systems reported tactile sensations sufficiently informative to guide object manipulation without visual feedback.

AI neural encoder models, including deep recurrent networks trained on simultaneous neural recording and tactile sensor data, learn the mapping from physical contact parameters to the multi-electrode stimulation patterns that most faithfully reproduce the corresponding natural neural responses [9]. This encoding problem is fundamentally ill-posed: the space of possible multi-electrode stimulation patterns is vastly larger than the space of natural neural responses, requiring AI optimization to find stimulation patterns within safe charge density limits that maximize perceptual fidelity. Reinforcement learning approaches in which the participant's reported sensory experience provides the reward signal enable personalized encoder optimization without requiring ground-truth neural recording during natural touch. Table 6.2 surveys different BCI sensory feedback modalities from scalp EEG with vibrotactile coupling through to optogenetic haptics detailing the interface site, AI architecture, and current clinical application or trial status for each. Figure 6.2 illustrates the complete BCI-haptic feedback architecture, tracing the signal pathway from prosthetic fingertip tactile sensors through AI encoding to sensory cortex or peripheral nerve stimulation and the patient's perceived tactile experience.

6.2.2   Peripheral Nerve Interfaces for Natural Touch

Peripheral nerve stimulation (PNS) interfaces electrodes implanted around or within the median, ulnar, or radial nerves of the residual limb and offers a less invasive alternative to cortical implants for haptic feedback restoration in amputees [4]. The transversal intrafascicular multichannel electrode (TIME) and the Utah Slanted Electrode Array (USEA) achieve selective activation of fascicles within the nerve, enabling spatial discrimination of sensory percepts across multiple digits. AI-driven stimulation parameter optimisation using Gaussian Process Regression to efficiently explore the high-dimensional pulse amplitude-width-frequency parameter space identifies the stimulation profiles that evoke the most naturalistic percepts for each individual patient within a practical clinical calibration session.

Closed-loop PNS systems continuously adjust stimulation parameters in response to real-time feedback from prosthetic tactile sensors and, where available, physiological

Table 6.2 Brain–computer interface sensory feedback modalities

BCI modality	Interface site	AI architecture	Clinical application and status
EEG + vibrotactile	Scalp (non-invasive)	CNN decoder + RL controller	Stroke motor rehab; commercially available systems
ECoG haptic feedback	Cortical surface (semi-inv.)	RNN spike decoder	Hand prosthesis touch restoration; Phase I/II trials
Intracortical microstimulation	S1 cortex (invasive)	Deep RL neural encoder	Dexterous prosthetic sensation; BrainGate/Neuralink trials
Peripheral nerve stimulation	Median/ulnar nerves	CNN tactile encoder	Amputee touch feedback; HAPTIX DARPA program
Spinal cord stimulation	Dorsal epidural	Closed-loop RL	Lower-limb sensory restoration in SCI; onward medical
Transcranial magnetic stimulation	Cortex (non-invasive)	Predictive pulse sequencer	Rehabilitation neuroplasticity induction; clinical trials
Optogenetic haptics (pre-clin.)	Sensory neurons	Light-pattern AI encoder	Precision mechanoreceptor activation; rodent models only

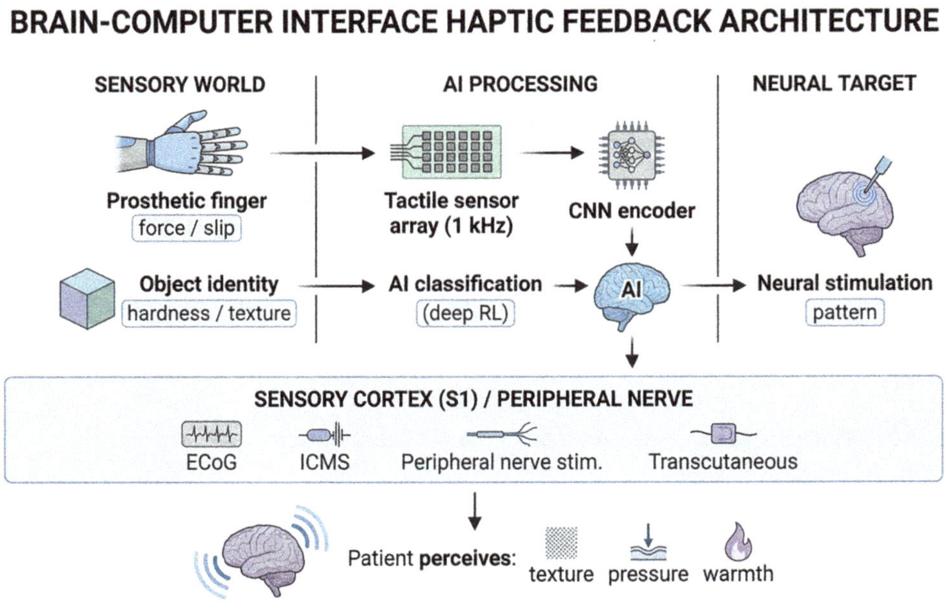

Fig. 6.2 Architecture of brain–computer interface haptic feedback system

biomarkers of neural adaptation (impedance spectroscopy of the neural interface). Longitudinal clinical studies of the HAPTIX programme (DARPA) demonstrated stable sensory percepts over 13 months of continuous implantation, with participants reporting improved prosthetic embodiment and reduced phantom limb pain suggesting that restoring peripheral sensory input suppresses the maladaptive cortical reorganization that underlies phantom pain [8].

6.2.3 Non-invasive BCI Approaches

For the large population of patients who cannot or will not accept invasive neural interfaces, non-invasive BCI approaches offer a pragmatic path to AI-haptic sensory enhancement. Transcranial magnetic stimulation (TMS) applied to sensory cortex can evoke tactile phosphenes—artificial sensations experienced without peripheral sensory input—that can be spatially steered by adjusting the TMS coil position and orientation [10]. AI systems that co-register TMS stimulation parameters with real-time EEG recordings of cortical state can deliver stimulation during optimal neural excitability windows identified from EEG oscillatory phase to maximize the signal-to-noise ratio of the evoked percept. While current TMS-haptic systems lack the spatial resolution and temporal precision of invasive interfaces, they are being actively explored for neuroplasticity induction in stroke rehabilitation, where the ability to deliver precisely timed somatosensory stimulation during voluntary movement attempts may accelerate motor recovery.

6.3   Soft Robotics and Next-Generation Prosthetics

The field of soft robotics which designs actuators, structures, and sensors from compliant, deformable materials rather than the rigid links and bearings of conventional robotics is converging with AI-haptic technology to produce the next generation of prosthetic and assistive devices [3]. Soft robotic prosthetics offer intrinsic safety advantages over rigid devices: a soft actuator that encounters unexpected resistance deforms rather than transmitting injurious forces; a pneumatically actuated finger collapses under excessive load rather than fracturing a fragile object or injuring a caregiver. These inherent compliance characteristics are particularly valuable in prosthetics, where devices must interact safely with fragile objects, human skin, and unpredictable environments.

6.3.1   Soft Actuator Technologies for Prosthetics

Several soft actuator technologies are approaching the performance levels required for dexterous prosthetic hands. Pneumatically actuated silicone fingers as used in the Soft Robotics Inc. gripper platform demonstrate grip forces of 5–20 N with inherently compliant grasping strategies that adapt to object geometry without complex sensing [3]. Shape memory alloy (SMA) actuators thin nickel-titanium wires that contract when electrically heated above their transition temperature offer muscle-like actuation in an extremely compact form factor, enabling prosthetic wrist rotation and finger articulation in a total device weight approaching that of a biological hand (approximately 400 g). Dielectric elastomer actuators (DEAs) polymer films that contract under applied electric field achieve high energy density actuation with silent operation, addressing a significant user experience limitation of pneumatic and SMA devices.

AI control of soft actuator prosthetics must address the unique challenge of highly nonlinear, history-dependent actuator dynamics: the force output of a pneumatic finger depends not only on current pressure but on the history of pressurization cycles, temperature, and cumulative material fatigue [11]. Physics-informed neural networks that incorporate the governing partial differential equations of soft material mechanics into their architecture generalize more effectively across operating conditions than data-driven approaches alone, reducing the data requirements for accurate actuator control model learning. Table 6.3 catalogues soft robotic and next-generation prosthetic innovations from pneumatic silicone actuators to stretchable electronic skin specifying the core technology, AI integration approach, and the advantage each offers over conventional rigid devices. Figure 6.3 presents the contrasting architectures of traditional and next-generation prosthetics side by side, showing how AI-controlled soft robotic systems with stretchable e-skin and neural stimulation feedback supersede the rigid, binary-state devices of today.

Table 6.3 Soft robotic and next-generation prosthetic innovations

Innovation	Core technology	AI integration	Advantages over conventional devices
Soft pneumatic actuators	Silicone + pneumatics	RL compliance control	Inherent safe human contact; no rigid failure modes
Dielectric elastomer actuators	Electro-active polymer	Neural network impedance	High energy density; silent; lightweight prosthetic fingers
Shape memory alloy drives	NiTi SMA wires	Predictive temperature control	Compact muscle-like actuation; prosthetic wrist rotation
Liquid crystal elastomers	Photo-responsive polymer	AI light-pattern actuation	Untethered soft robotic finger; wireless activation
Bio-hybrid muscle actuators	Living skeletal muscle	Bioelectronic AI control	Organic force generation; self-repair capability
Granular jamming skin	Coffee-ground matrix	AI stiffness mapping	Variable-compliance prosthetic palm; adaptive grasping
Stretchable electronics skin	Nanomaterial sensors	CNN multi-modal fusion	Distributed tactile sensing matching human fingertip density

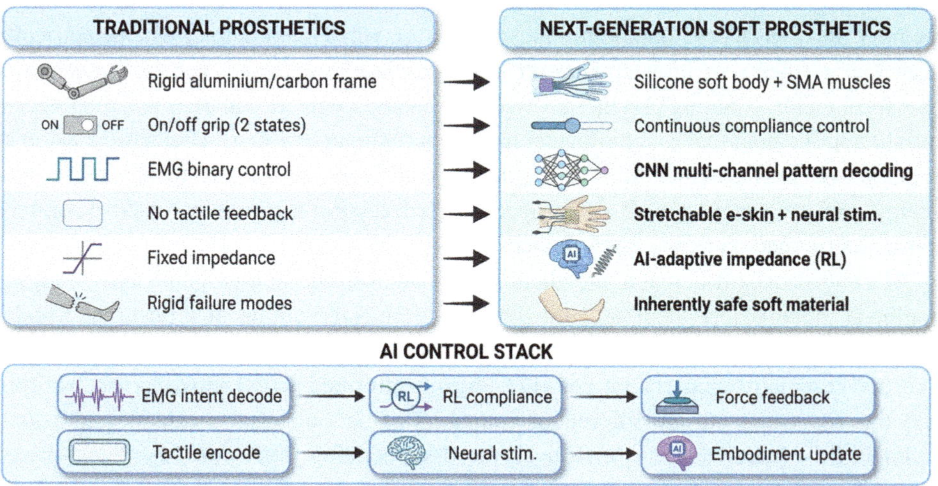

Fig. 6.3 Architecture of soft robotics and next-generation prosthetics

6.3.2   Bio-hybrid Actuators and Living Prosthetics

The most radical frontier of prosthetic actuation is the bio-hybrid approach: devices powered by living skeletal muscle tissue cultured on artificial scaffolds and controlled through bioelectronic AI interfaces [3]. Biological muscle offers unmatched energy density, self-repair capability, and seamless electrophysiological interfacing with the nervous system properties that no purely artificial actuator has yet replicated. Proof-of-concept bio-hybrid robotic fingers have demonstrated controllable flexion and extension powered by cultured muscle sheets in response to electrical stimulation. AI bioelectronic controllers that read motor intent from residual nerve EMG signals and translate them to spatially and temporally patterned electrical stimulation of the muscle sheet represent a closed-loop biological actuation system with potential for organic prosthetic integration.

The regulatory and ethical dimensions of bio-hybrid prosthetics are substantially more complex than those of purely artificial devices: living tissue components raise questions about device lifecycle (cell viability maintenance), sterility, personalization (patient-derived vs. allogenic cells), and the moral status of sentient tissue incorporated into a machine [12]. These questions require proactive engagement between developers, ethicists, regulatory bodies, and patient communities before clinical translation proceeds.

6.4   Smart Hospitals and Digital Healthcare Ecosystems

The individual AI-haptic systems examined throughout this book— such as surgical robots, rehabilitation exoskeletons, and haptic telemedicine platforms— are progressively being embedded within a broader digital hospital ecosystem in which interconnected AI systems share patient data, coordinate clinical workflows, and continuously improve through collective learning across the institution [13]. The smart hospital of the near future integrates AI-haptic technologies not as isolated point solutions but as components of a coherent, interoperable digital infrastructure built on patient digital twins, federated AI platforms, and real-time IoMT sensor networks.

6.4.1   Patient Digital Twins

A patient digital twin is a continuously updated computational model of an individual patient integrating anatomical imaging, genomic data, physiological monitoring, treatment history, and real-world sensor data that enables personalized simulation of clinical interventions before they are applied to the physical patient [14]. For AI-haptic surgery, the digital twin provides the patient-specific virtual environment in which the surgical team rehearses the procedure, the AI tissue classification model is pre-trained on the patient's specific tissue biomechanics, and surgical trajectories are optimized before the first incision. Physics-informed neural networks trained on the patient's imaging data predict tissue deformation, cutting forces, and bleeding risk with a level of patient-specificity that population-average models cannot approach.

Digital twins also serve as the data substrate for post-market surveillance and continuous improvement: by comparing the simulated procedure outcome with the actual intraoperative haptic data, manufacturers and clinicians can identify systematic discrepancies that indicate model limitations, patient-subgroup performance degradation, or emerging safety signals providing a real-world evidence generation mechanism that far exceeds the capability of conventional adverse event reporting. Table 6.4 maps smart hospital ecosystem layers from the digital twin platform and AR surgical navigation to AI rehabilitation wards and robotic pharmacy describing the technology, AI-haptic role, and expected clinical outcome at each layer. Figure 6.4 illustrates the full digital ecosystem architecture, connecting the operating theatre, rehabilitation ward, and outpatient or remote care domains through a unified hospital AI platform and digital twin core, with cloud population analytics above.

6.4.2 Augmented Reality and Haptic-AR Co-registration

The convergence of AI-haptic systems with augmented reality surgical navigation represents one of the most clinically exciting near-term developments in the smart operating theatre [15]. AR headsets (Microsoft HoloLens 2, Magic Leap 2) overlay pre-operative imaging data— tumour boundaries, vascular anatomy, and nerve trajectories— directly onto the surgeon's visual field in real time, creating a spatially registered anatomical guidance system. When this visual AR overlay is coupled with AI-haptic virtual fixtures— force barriers that physically resist tool entry into AR-designated danger zones— the system provides simultaneous visual and tactile anatomical guidance. The surgeon sees the danger boundary through the AR overlay and feels it resists their instrument approach.

Achieving accurate haptic—AR co-registration in the deforming intraoperative environment—where tissue displacement is due to retraction, breathing, and cardiac motion continuously invalidates pre-operative geometric models require real-time AI model updating. Deformable image registration networks that predict tissue deformation from

Table 6.4 Smart hospital digital ecosystem layers

Ecosystem layer	Technology	AI-haptic role	Clinical outcome
Digital twin platform	Patient-specific simulation	Pre-operative haptic rehearsal	Reduced intraoperative complications by procedure planning
AR surgical navigation	HoloLens 2/Magic Leap	Haptic-AR co-registration	Overlay anatomy on live tissue with haptic boundary alerts
Autonomous surgical robots	Vision + force AI	Supervised autonomous suturing	Consistent knot tension regardless of surgeon fatigue
AI triage and diagnosis	Multi-modal sensing	Haptic palpation remote triage	Remote ED assessment with tactile palpation fidelity
Predictive ward management	IoMT + NLP EHR mining	Haptic alert wearables for staff	Proactive patient deterioration alerts to nursing staff
Robotic pharmacy/ logistics	AMR + grippers	Force-sensitive drug handling	Zero-dispensing-error robotic pharmacy with haptic QC
AI rehabilitation ward	Full-room sensor mesh	Adaptive haptic therapy scheduling	24/7 AI-managed rehabilitation intensity optimisation

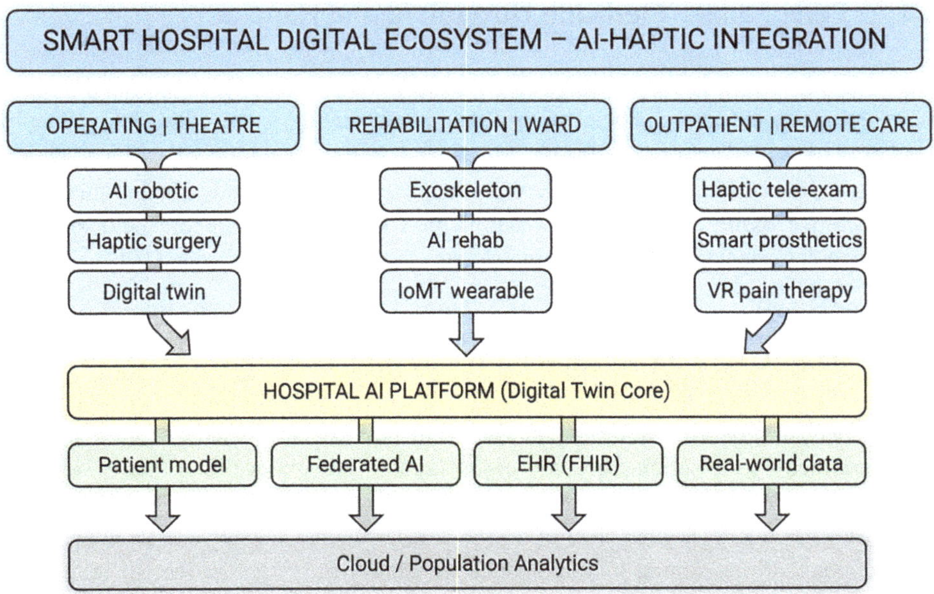

Fig. 6.4 Smart hospital digital ecosystem

sparse intraoperative sensor measurements update the AR geometric model and haptic virtual fixture boundaries at surgical frame rates (30–60 Hz), maintaining co-registration accuracy below the perceptual threshold for co-registration error [5].

6.4.3   Autonomous Surgical Systems

The long-term trajectory of AI-haptic surgical systems points toward increasing degrees of task-level autonomy robots that not only assist the surgeon but perform defined procedural subtasks independently under human supervision [15]. The Smart Tissue Autonomous Robot (STAR) demonstrated autonomous laparoscopic intestinal anastomosis in porcine models, outperforming human surgeons on consistency of suture placement and anastomotic leak rate using a combination of computer vision, force sensing, and pre-programmed motion planning. Future autonomous surgical systems will integrate AI-haptic force control as a primary safety mechanism: the robot's haptic sensing layer provides the physical feedback that enables compliant, tissue-respecting motion even when visual guidance is insufficient.

6.5   Personalized Medicine Through AI and Haptics

Personalized medicine, the tailoring of clinical interventions to the specific biological, psychological, and social characteristics of individual patients, is one of the defining ambitions of twenty-first century healthcare. AI-haptic systems are uniquely positioned to contribute to this ambition because they both generate highly individual patient data (intraoperative tissue force profiles, rehabilitation kinematics, pain threshold measurements) and can adapt their behaviour in response to that data in real time [10].

6.5.1   Multi-Omics Integration for Tissue Biomechanics Prediction

The mechanical properties of biological tissue stiffness, viscosity, and fracture toughness are determined by the composition and organisation of the extracellular matrix, which is in turn regulated by the genomic, transcriptomic, and proteomic profile of the tissue. Graph neural networks trained on multi-omics datasets linked to ex vivo tissue mechanical measurements are beginning to demonstrate the ability to predict patient-specific tissue biomechanical properties from pre-operative genomic profiling enabling AI-haptic surgical systems to initialize patient-specific force rendering models before the first intraoperative contact [14]. This approach is particularly valuable for connective tissue disorders (Ehlers-Danlos syndrome and Marfan syndrome) in which tissue mechanical properties deviate markedly from population averages, and where the use of standard-parameterized haptic force limits could lead to inadvertent tissue damage.

Table 6.5 structures personalization dimensions from tissue biomechanics and neurological profile to prosthetic embodiment and surgical learning curve specifying the data source, AI method, and resulting haptic system adaptation for each. Figure 6.5 presents the personalized medicine pipeline, showing how multi-modal patient data inputs flow through the patient digital twin to produce adaptive haptic system parameters governing surgical force profiles, rehabilitation intensity, prosthetic feedback, and pain analgesia.

6.5.2   Neurological Phenotyping for Sensory Optimization

Individual differences in somatosensory processing including cutaneous tactile thresholds, two-point discrimination, vibration frequency sensitivity, and thermal detection exhibit substantial population variance driven by age, sex, neurological health, and genetic factors [4]. Quantitative sensory testing (QST) protocols that characterize an individual's sensory profile across multiple modalities can parameterize AI-haptic rendering models to deliver stimuli matched to that individual's perceptual thresholds and preferences. For rehabilitation haptics, personalized vibrotactile frequency selection matching the stimulation frequency to the patient's specific optimal vibration frequency for proprioceptive substitution

Table 6.5 Personalized medicine dimensions

Personalization dimension	Data source	AI method	Haptic system adaptation
Tissue biomechanics	Pre-op CT/MRI + ex vivo data	Physics-informed neural network	Patient-specific force rendering profile for surgery
Neurological profile	fMRI + EEG + psychophysics	Bayesian personalization model	Optimized vibrotactile frequency for sensory threshold
Motor recovery trajectory	Longitudinal kinematic data	LSTM trajectory predictor	Adaptive rehabilitation assistance level per session
Genomic-haptic correlation	WGS + tissue stiffness assay	Graph neural network	Predict tissue properties from genomic connective tissue markers
Pain sensitivity phenotype	QST + patient-reported outcomes	Gaussian process regression	Personalized TENS/ vibration analgesia dose-response curve
Prosthetic embodiment	fMRI + body ownership illusion test	RL embodiment optimizer	Personalized sensory feedback mapping for phantom ownership
Surgical learning curve	Simulation performance history	Continual learning model	Adaptive surgical haptic guidance intensity per trainee level

has been shown to improve motor learning rates by 23% compared to fixed-frequency stimulation.

6.5.3   Longitudinal Adaptation and Predictive Personalization

The most powerful form of AI-haptic personalization is longitudinal: systems that accumulate patient-specific data across multiple clinical encounters and continuously refine their personalization models. Continual learning architectures that update patient-specific haptic parameter profiles after each surgical procedure, rehabilitation session, or prosthetic use period while preserving generalized population-level knowledge through elastic weight consolidation enable haptic systems that become progressively better calibrated to each patient over time [16]. Predictive personalization models that forecast how a patient's sensory thresholds, motor capacity, or tissue biomechanics will evolve over the course of a disease or recovery trajectory enable proactive adjustment of haptic system parameters anticipating the patient's future needs rather than reacting to observed performance degradation.

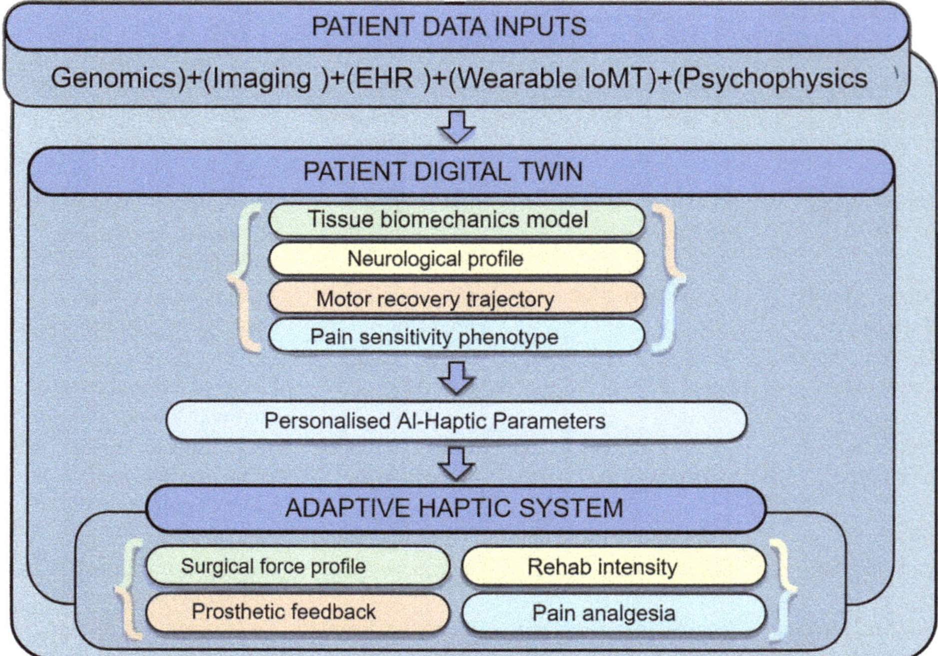

Fig. 6.5 Personalized medicine pipeline through AI-haptic integration

6.6   Research Directions and Innovation Opportunities

The AI-haptic healthcare field stands at an inflection point: foundational technologies are proven, clinical applications are emerging from trials, and the regulatory frameworks are beginning to mature. The research agenda for the next 15 years must simultaneously push the technological frontier toward greater capability and accessibility while building the clinical evidence base, safety engineering infrastructure, and global equity mechanisms that responsible deployment requires [12, 17].

6.6.1   Foundation Models for Haptic Intelligence

Large language models (GPT-4, Claude, Gemini) have demonstrated that pre-training on vast diverse datasets produces general-purpose AI systems that can be efficiently fine-tuned for specific downstream tasks. An analogous 'haptic foundation model' pre-trained on a large, diverse corpus of haptic sensor data from surgical, rehabilitation, prosthetic, and telemedicine applications would encode general representations of tissue mechanics, tactile textures, and human motor interaction that could be fine-tuned with minimal data for new clinical applications [18, 19]. Building such a model requires coordinated international data collection infrastructure standardized haptic sensor formats, data annotation ontologies, and federated training protocols representing a major research coordination challenge that mirrors the genomics data commons initiatives of the past decade.

6.6.2   The Haptic Internet

The haptic internet, a global network infrastructure capable of transmitting tactile information with the round-trip latency, reliability, and fidelity required for real-time haptic interaction, would transform telemedicine by enabling physical examination, surgical tele-operation, and haptic rehabilitation at any geographic distance [20]. The fundamental engineering challenge is the round-trip latency requirement: human tactile perception becomes aware of delays greater than approximately 1 ms during active manipulation tasks, implying that haptic internet transmission must reduce effective latency below this threshold through a combination of physical network improvements (6G sub-terahertz links) and AI predictive rendering. The AI predictor must model the remote physical environment well enough to render plausible haptic responses locally while true sensor data is in transit, a form of distributed digital twin computation.

6G network technology, with target round-trip latencies below 1 ms and data rates above 1 Tbps, provides the physical layer foundation for the haptic internet [20]. Quantum key distribution (QKD) secured communication channels will address the data sovereignty and cybersecurity requirements for transmitting sensitive patient haptic data across international network infrastructure. The WHO's proposed Digital Health Accord analogous to existing pandemic preparedness agreements could provide the international governance framework for haptic internet access, ensuring that low- and middle-income countries are not excluded from the clinical benefits of haptic telemedicine.

6.6.3   Open Science and Global Research Collaboration

Accelerating progress in AI-haptic healthcare requires open science infrastructure: shared datasets, open-source AI models, and collaborative clinical trial networks that span income settings and geographic regions [12, 21]. The Open Haptics data initiative modelled on the Human Connectome Project and UK Biobank should aggregate standardized haptic procedure data from surgical, rehabilitation, prosthetic, and telemedicine applications across global clinical sites, with equitable data access policies enabling researchers in all countries to contribute to and benefit from the collective knowledge base. Precompetitive consortia involving medical device manufacturers, academic medical centres, and patient organisations can align commercial and public health incentives around shared technical standards and evidence generation frameworks.

6.7   Vision for the Future of Human–Machine Collaboration

The technology landscape examined in this chapter points toward a future of AI-haptic healthcare characterized not by the replacement of human clinicians with autonomous machines, but by a progressively deeper and more productive collaboration between human intelligence and artificial intelligence—each contributing capabilities the other lacks, mediated by haptic interfaces that make this collaboration tactile, intuitive, and immediate [22]. This collaborative vision is not merely a technological projection; it is a normative commitment about the kind of medicine we wish to create.

6.7.1   Complementary Intelligence Architecture

Human clinical intelligence and AI-haptic system intelligence are deeply complementary rather than competitive. Human surgeons bring strategic reasoning—the ability to recognize an unexpected anatomical variant, revise the operative plan, and communicate a decision to the theatre team in seconds—that AI systems operating on pre-trained models cannot replicate for novel situations. AI-haptic systems bring computational capabilities that no human can match: continuous processing of 1000 sensor channels at 1 kHz, fatigue-free consistency across an eight-hour operating list and recall of every procedure performed on every patient in the training dataset [10]. The optimal clinical outcome is achieved when human strategic intelligence directs AI computational power through an intuitive haptic interface, not when either operates alone.

6.7.2   Tactile Medicine as a New Clinical Discipline

The convergence of AI and haptic technology gives rise to what may be understood as a new clinical discipline: tactile medicine, the systematic use of engineered touch, mediated by AI-haptic systems, as both a diagnostic and therapeutic modality [23]. Just as interventional radiology emerged from the convergence of imaging and catheter technology to create a new clinical specialty, tactile medicine will draw together surgical robotics, rehabilitation engineering, prosthetics, BCI neuroscience, and telemedicine haptics into a coherent clinical and scientific identity. This discipline will require new training programmes, new professional competency frameworks, new clinical performance metrics, and new research methodologies in investments that the medical community and educational institutions must begin planning now.

6.7.3 Ethical Stewardship as a Continuing Obligation

The responsible innovation framework established in Chap. 5 is not a regulatory threshold to be crossed at the point of product launch, but a continuing obligation that must be discharged throughout the lifecycle of AI-haptic healthcare technologies. As capabilities expand—as autonomous surgical systems perform more complex tasks, BCI-haptic interfaces penetrate deeper into the nervous system, and digital twins accumulate increasingly intimate patient data— the ethical stakes increase in proportion [12]. The medical community, technology developers, patients, and regulators must maintain an active, adaptive ethical dialogue that anticipates these expanding stakes and updates governance frameworks before harm occurs rather than in response to it.

The long-term vision for AI-haptic healthcare is ultimately a humanistic one: technology that extends the reach of skilled clinical care to every patient who needs it, regardless of geography, wealth, or disability, gives the surgeon's hands greater sensitivity than biology alone provides, restores the sense of touch to those who have lost it, and enables a physiotherapist in one country to guide a rehabilitation patient in another through the same haptic channel they would use face-to-face [17]. Realizing this vision requires not only the engineering excellence and scientific rigour documented throughout this book, but the moral commitment to ensure that the benefits of AI-haptic innovation reach all of humanity.

6.8 Summary

This chapter explores the future trends and innovations in AI-driven haptic healthcare, focusing on emerging technologies, their integration into clinical applications, and the ethical considerations for responsible innovation. It examines advancements in haptic interfaces, such as mid-air ultrasonic displays, soft microfluidic skins, and neuromorphic chips, which promise to enhance tactile interaction in healthcare. The chapter highlights the transformative potential of brain–computer interfaces (BCIs) for restoring natural touch and sensory feedback, as well as the development of soft robotics and bio-hybrid actuators for next-generation prosthetics. It discusses the integration of AI-haptic systems into smart hospital ecosystems, emphasizing patient digital twins, augmented reality surgical navigation, and autonomous surgical systems. The chapter also delves into personalized medicine, leveraging multi-omics data and AI to tailor haptic systems to individual patients. Finally, it outlines research directions, including the creation of haptic foundation models, the development of a global haptic internet, and the establishment of tactile medicine as a new clinical discipline, all underpinned by ethical stewardship to ensure equitable access and responsible deployment of these technologies.

References

1. Pacchierotti, C., Sinclair, S., Solazzi, M., Frisoli, A., Hayward, V., & Prattichizzo, D. (2017). Wearable haptic systems for the fingertip and the hand: Taxonomy, review, and perspectives. *IEEE Transactions on Haptics, 10*(4), 580–600.
2. Shanmugam, M., Venusamy, K., Subin, S., Srivatsan, S., & Kumar, N. (2023, March). A comprehensive review of haptic gloves: Advances, challenges, and future directions. In *2023 Second International Conference on Electronics and Renewable Systems (ICEARS)* (pp. 227–233). IEEE.
3. Rus, D., & Tolley, M. T. (2015). Design, fabrication and control of soft robots. *Nature, 521*(7553), 467–475.
4. Johansson, R. S., & Flanagan, J. R. (2009). Coding and use of tactile signals from the fingertips in object manipulation tasks. *Nature Reviews Neuroscience, 10*(5), 345–359.
5. Laycock, S. D., & Day, A. M. (2007, March). A survey of haptic rendering techniques. *Computer Graphics Forum, 26*(1), 50–65.
6. Hochberg, L. R., Bacher, D., Jarosiewicz, B., Masse, N. Y., Simeral, J. D., Vogel, J., et al. (2012). Reach and grasp by people with tetraplegia using a neurally controlled robotic arm. *Nature, 485*(7398), 372–375.
7. Collinger, J. L., Wodlinger, B., Downey, J. E., Wang, W., Tyler-Kabara, E. C., Weber, D. J., et al. (2013). High-performance neuroprosthetic control by an individual with tetraplegia. *The Lancet, 381*(9866), 557–564.
8. Bensmaia, S. J., & Miller, L. E. (2014). Restoring sensorimotor function through intracortical interfaces: Progress and looming challenges. *Nature Reviews Neuroscience, 15*(5), 313–325.
9. Shenoy, K. V., & Carmena, J. M. (2014). Combining decoder design and neural adaptation in brain-machine interfaces. *Neuron, 84*(4), 665–680.
10. Topol, E. J. (2019). High-performance medicine: The convergence of human and artificial intelligence. *Nature Medicine, 25*(1), 44–56.
11. Sutton, R. S., & Barto, A. G. (1998). *Reinforcement learning: An introduction* (pp. 9–11). MIT Press.
12. World Health Organization. (2021). *Ethics and governance of artificial intelligence for health.* WHO Press. https://www.who.int/publications/i/item/9789240029200
13. Riek, L. D. (2017). Healthcare robotics. *Communications of the ACM, 60*(11), 68–78.
14. Raissi, M., Perdikaris, P., & Karniadakis, G. E. (2019). Physics-informed neural networks: A deep learning framework for solving forward and inverse problems involving nonlinear partial differential equations. *Journal of Computational Physics, 378*, 686–707.
15. Zemmar, A., Lozano, A. M., & Nelson, B. J. (2020). The rise of robots in surgical environments during COVID-19. *Nature Machine Intelligence, 2*(10), 566–572.
16. Finn, C., Abbeel, P., & Levine, S. (2017, July). Model-agnostic meta-learning for fast adaptation of deep networks. In *International conference on machine learning* (pp. 1126–1135). PMLR.
17. United Nations. (2015). *Transforming our world: The 2030 Agenda for Sustainable Development.* UN General Assembly Resolution A/RES/70/1.
18. LeCun, Y., Bengio, Y., & Hinton, G. (2015). Deep learning. *Nature, 521*(7553), 436–444.
19. Vaswani, A., Shazeer, N., Parmar, N., Uszkoreit, J., Jones, L., Gomez, A. N., et al. (2017). Attention is all you need. *Advances in Neural Information Processing Systems, 30*.
20. Shi, W., Cao, J., Zhang, Q., Li, Y., & Xu, L. (2016). Edge computing: Vision and challenges. *IEEE Internet of Things Journal, 3*(5), 637–646.
21. McMahan, B., Moore, E., Ramage, D., Hampson, S., & y Arcas, B. A. (2017, April). Communication-efficient learning of deep networks from decentralized data. In *Artificial intelligence and statistics* (pp. 1273–1282).

22. Haddadin, S., & Croft, E. (2016). Physical human–robot interaction. In *Springer handbook of robotics* (pp. 1835–1874). Springer.
23. Okamura, A. M. (2009). Haptic feedback in robot-assisted minimally invasive surgery. *Current Opinion in Urology, 19*(1), 102–107.

GPSR Compliance
The European Union's (EU) General Product Safety Regulation (GPSR) is a set
of rules that requires consumer products to be safe and our obligations to
ensure this.

If you have any concerns about our products, you can contact us on

ProductSafety@springernature.com

In case Publisher is established outside the EU, the EU authorized
representative is:

Springer Nature Customer Service Center GmbH
Europaplatz 3
69115 Heidelberg, Germany